Fitness at 40, 50, 60 And Beyond

Michael Spitzer

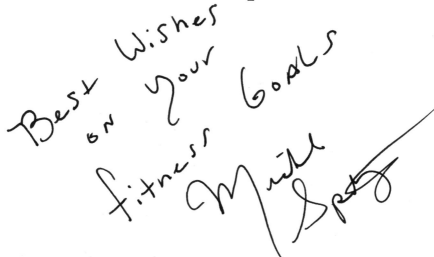

Fitness at 40, 50, 60 And Beyond

Michael Spitzer

High Point

HighPoint Products – Weston, Florida
2014

Written by Michael Spitzer
Edited by Michael Höhne and Angela Werner
Cover Art by Rich DiSilvio - Digital Vista
Interior Design by Angela Werner, Höhne-Werner Design
Gym Photography by Evelyn Robles - evelyn.robles@live.com
Home Photography by Glenna Spitzer
Additional Photographs and Images used by licensed agreement with Can Stock Photo and Shutterstock.

Published by HighPoint Products
4581 Weston Road #297
Weston, Florida 33331
www.highpointproducts.com

Printed in the United States of America

First Edition - January 2014
First Printing - January 2014

Library of Congress Control Number: 2013938427

ISBN-13: 978-0-9890348-0-7

This book is not intended to be a substitute for professional medical advice, diagnosis, counseling, or treatment.

The contents of "Fitness at 40, 50, 60 and Beyond" are for informational purposes only.

This book includes information from a wide range of sources and collected from many personal experiences. It is sold with the understanding that neither the author nor publisher is engaged in providing any legal, medical, or psychological advice.

As it is impossible to know the individual health history of everyone who may read this book, it is highly advisable that you discuss the contents with your doctor to determine if these exercise routines and diet guidelines are suitable for your own personal condition.

Use of the programs within this book is at the sole risk and choice of the reader.

Contents

Chapter One

Does The World Really Need
Another Book About Getting Fit?

Why This Book Was Written

This book was not originally my idea.

In fact, if you had asked my opinion several years ago, I would have said the world already has more than enough books, magazines, and infomercials dedicated to the goal of helping people lose weight and feel better. As it turns out, I was wrong. There is an entire portion of our population that has been largely overlooked by the mainstream fitness craze. However, I did not make that discovery on my own.

This book is in your hands because dozens of people kept telling me: *Your advice and routines have done more for me than anything I have tried in the past. You should write a book.* When people started urging me to write a manual focusing on the special challenges and needs of people over age 40, I began to wonder why, with all the existing material on the market, there was a perceived need for such a book.

The Fitness Industry Caters To the Young

Next time you visit a supermarket or bookstore, take a look at the magazine rack. No doubt you will find at least half a dozen magazines featuring models on the cover who resemble Mr. Universe, or, a perfect example of the feminine physique clad in a bikini containing less fabric than a dinner napkin. Almost certainly, these cover models will be under the age of 30.

Now grab one of those same magazines off the shelf and take a quick read through the pages. Personally, I have enjoyed reading and learning about exercise and fitness from these magazines since the 1970s, but they tend to be more dedicated to youthful hardcore training. There is plenty of great information to be found between the covers of these publications, but unless you are genetically gifted and using chemical enhancement, they often demonstrate a level of development that is un-obtainable to 99% of the general public.

The objective of this book is to extract the best fitness information of the past 50 years into a single reference source providing superior advice and benefits for older individuals. The information in the pages that follow is designed to give the best "bang for the buck" in terms of ob-taining results, while taking into consideration special concerns of joint health, slowing metabolism, hormonal changes, and other challenges for those well into the second half of life.

Despite All the Information Available, People Continue to Minimize Benefits and Maximize the Risk of Injury

Every day at gyms around the world, you will witness people unknowingly doing things that place them at risk of injury. This improper use of equipment and/or faulty body mechanics can potentially damage joints, tendons, and ligaments while failing to properly exercise the targeted muscle fibers.

A common example of this phenomenon looks much like the following example:

An individual will place ten or more large weight plates on the leg press machine. The leg press machine is designed to exercise the muscles of the leg. Specifically, the quadriceps muscle is the part of the leg most heavily targeted with this exercise, with benefit also being shared by the hamstrings, calves, and buttocks. With ten or more plates loaded on this specific machine, the total weight can exceed 500 pounds.

They will then sit in the machine, place their feet on the platform, and press this massive weight no more than 1–3 inches at the point where the knee is only moving from a slightly bent to straight and locked position (Photo 1.1).

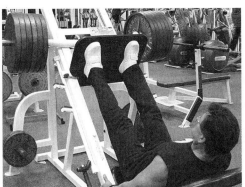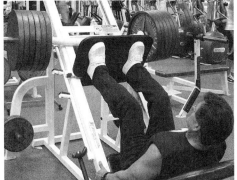

(Photo 1.1) Improper Limited Range of Motion: Knees barely bending during a leg press exercise.

What is really happening here? The muscles of the leg are receiving almost no stimulation or benefit from this short, limited movement. The knee joint is being subjected to a large amount of leveraged force near the end of its natural range of motion.

Think about the simple action of getting up from a seated position. Where is the motion the hardest? Where is the motion the easiest?

When you first start to stand up, you feel the front of your legs doing most of the work. But as you finish the motion and straighten your legs, you no longer feel much work being done by your leg muscles.

In a standing position, your straightened knees and bones carry the majority of your weight. Because of simple mechanics and the hinge structure of the knee, leverage is working to your advantage during the last few inches as the leg straightens to a standing position.

This same principle is demonstrated by the difference in difficulty you experience when walking up stairs as compared to walking along a flat surface. In the first case, your legs must bend approximately 90 degrees as they move upwards to the next step. In the latter case, your legs barely bend and very little effort is felt in the upper leg.

In our example, the individual has selected an excessively heavy weight that the knee joint can just barely handle in its most leveraged position of being nearly straight.

However, if they would try to raise and lower this weight through a full range of motion such as the leg would travel in the natural act of sitting or squatting, they would likely get crushed and folded like a pretzel beneath the sliding platform.

The goal for everyone, but even more importantly for those with some age behind them, is to strengthen the muscles and connective tissue, but protect the joints.

Performing weight resistance exercises in a manner that allows the muscle to work in a full and natural range of functional motion is vital to developing strength, protecting joints from injury, and allowing one to remain active much longer than the average sedentary citizen.

In the chapters describing the exercise routines you will be performing, we will cover in detail not only the "how," but also the "why" certain exercises are performed in the manner being demonstrated. You will learn the proper equipment and form to be used when performing both weight resistance and cardiovascular exercise.

Some Trainers Are Excellent, Others Are Too Busy Scoping Out the Meat Market

Many people feel a bit intimidated by the idea of joining a gym. For those with no prior experience or instruction, the variety of machines and wide variety of options can seem overwhelming.

Upon joining a commercial gym, many people will enlist the aid of a personal trainer. Personalized training is frequently offered at many larger establishments, with the trainers being certified by an organization such as (but not limited to) those listed below:

ACE – American Council on Exercise
ISSA – International Sports Sciences Association
NFPT – National Association of Personal Trainers
NASM – National Academy of Sports Medicine

A personal trainer who takes a genuine interest in your goals, structures a program specific to your needs, and is attentive during the training sessions can be a great boost for some people when first getting started.

However, there is another type of trainer seen far too often in the gym and fitness business today. These trainers are easy to spot. They are the guys telling a client to continue doing more repetitions of an exercise while not even watching them. Instead they are staring at the pretty young girl with the tight pants or obvious cleavage at the other end of the gym floor.

If this scenario sounds familiar and brought a grin to your face, you are by no means alone. Each time I have used this example, somebody in the group I am speaking with has cried out, "Exactly!"

While I would never discourage a person from paying for the services of a qualified and attentive personal trainer, this book should allow you to accomplish your goals independently and on your own terms.

There is a great sense of accomplishment in summoning forth your own motivation to research a topic, apply the information learned, and see your ambitions become reality.

Many People over Age 50 Missed the Knowledge of the Fitness Revolution

The mid 1970s through early 1980s is often considered the era when our modern fitness revolution came into existence. Before this time, the concepts behind exercise and nutrition were understood, but not yet widely accepted by the general population. In fact, prior to the 1977 film *Pumping Iron* starring Arnold Schwarzenegger, popular mainstream opinion of weight training was that it was a niche activity reserved for specialized athletes, muscle-bound freaks, or the very vain.

Not only were the benefits of weight resistance training largely misunderstood by the general population, but dietary principles were entrenched more in the traditions of Western living and less in the actual biological needs and functioning of the human body.

Some habits are hard to break. Even today with all that has been learned, the idea of three full course meals per day, with the evening dinner often being the largest, is still ingrained in our society. Even more so, there persists a misunderstanding regarding the primary nutritional components (Protein, Carbohydrates, and Fats) as well as the varied vitamins and minerals.

For example, several years ago a certain well known "Low Carbohydrate—High Protein" diet was the hot trend in America. People on this diet were avoiding bread, noodles, rice, oatmeal, or any form of carbohydrate as much as possible. At this same time they were eating

1: Does The World Really Need Another Book About Getting Fit?

substantial amounts of bacon, hamburger, sausage, and other meats. It was common during this time to hear cautionary tales regarding the risks of a "high protein diet."

Here is the irony. This infamous diet plan was not actually a high protein diet as much as it was a high fat diet. In this case, there was confusion over how much protein a food source contained as compared to the fat content.

Have you ever heard a person comment, "I eat peanut butter, so I get plenty of protein"? This is a perfect example of the misunderstanding that exists in our society as to the nutritional composition of common foods.

2 tablespoons of a typical name brand peanut butter contains:

17 grams of fat
6 grams of carbohydrates (50% of which is sugar)
7 grams of protein

A substantial portion of these fats come from hydrogenated oils.

Natural peanut butter is in fact a healthy food choice, as we will see later in the chapter on nutrition. But it is valued for the healthy fats it provides more than for its protein content. I refer here to natural peanut butter which has very few ingredients other than peanuts and salt. Truly natural peanut butter will NOT contain hydrogenated oils, sugar, or corn syrup.

By the way, some brands of peanut butter claim to be natural while also proudly proclaiming they need no stirring. This ability to keep the peanut butter from separating is accomplished by the addition of palm oil.

While it is technically accurate to refer to palm oil as a natural ingredient, this can be a little misleading. Palm oil is a naturally occurring but highly saturated vegetable fat. In fact, it is one of the few vegetable fats to possess this characteristic. Research conducted since the 1970s and as recently as 2006 indicate palm oil may have adverse effects on blood lipids and cholesterol values very similar to other trans-fats.

This brief discussion of peanut butter and palm oil is only introduced here as an example of what you can expect to learn in the pages to follow. The chapter on diet and nutrition may have you looking at food and nutrition quite differently than you did in the past.

What You Can Expect To Learn and Accomplish in the Pages that Follow

At the beginning of this chapter, I stated there have been volumes written over the years about diet, exercise, and weight loss.

Much less has been written about these topics as they apply specifically to people on the high side of 40. Most people don't have the time to undergo exhaustive research, decipher tons of articles, scrutinize conflicting data, or gamble money on questionable television infomercial products in a quest to find honest information to meet their goals.

This book is not intended to be a lengthy tome of fitness theory or simplistic motivational pep talk. Instead it is designed to be a distillation and summary of all the years of research that has come before it, combined and presented in an easy to digest format that will give you more functional fitness knowledge than 98% of the general population.

The information in this book, combined with your own personal dedication, will allow you to:

- Lose Weight and Decrease Body Fat
- Improve Muscle Size and Strength
- Boost Your Base Level Metabolism
- Improve Energy Levels and Vitality
- Look and Feel Years Younger
- Potentially Decrease Your Reliance on Medications

- Decrease Joint Pain and Improve Flexibility
- Improve Sexual Function
- Reduce Risk of Diabetes, Heart Attack, and Strokes
- Lower Stress Levels and Depression Symptoms
- Live Longer (with a better quality of life)

Bottom line, this book provides a clearly explained and proven recipe to improve your health, fitness, and function at 40, 50, 60, and beyond.

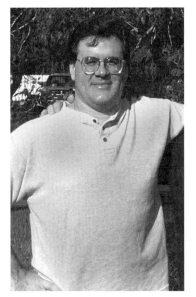 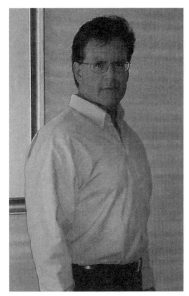

(Photo 1.2) The author unhealthy at age 35, and a new man at age 50 following the guidelines set forth in this book.

Chapter Two

Forty Is No Longer Over the Hill

Assuming We Live a Little Smarter

There was a time not too long ago when the accepted mindset was that once we reached 40 years of age, we were "over the hill." The best one could expect was to try to accept an inevitable decline down a sharp slope into the frailties of old age.

Looking back, it may at first seem this mindset was indeed accurate. After all, old photographs of family members often show a person who appears older than we know them to be by today's standards. To be sure, in today's youth-oriented culture, some of the change we see in people's appearances as compared to yesteryear can be attributed to hair coloring, plastic surgery, Botox injections, or other techniques. But there is more to it than that.

In the past, it seems many people lived their lives according to a self-fulfilling prophecy. Since the prevailing thought process was that it is "all downhill" after age 40, most people subconsciously adapted their lifestyles to match this mentality. Gaining weight was simply accepted as an unavoidable change of life. Loss of muscle tone, aches and pains, and cutting back on once-loved activities was considered part of the normal aging process.

Here is the harsh truth. The average person was short-changing themselves. They were "going to seed," resigning themselves to a reduced level of energy and fitness, too early in life.

Are you ready for another harsh truth? Many people today are still living their lives according to this inaccurate and outdated mindset.

Modern research has revealed many interesting facts regarding aging, and dispelled a series of long held beliefs, for example:

- Even those who have been exercising regularly for years can still add **new** muscle size and strength into their late 50s.

- Time and time again, it has been shown that people who remain active and have a lifestyle which combines reasonable eating with some form of cardiovascular and weight resistance exercise are more mobile and perform better into their 70s than do sedentary people in their 30s.

- Toning and strengthening of existing muscle fibers can be attained at any age, even well into your 80s.

- Once they begin a structured program, persons who have not been physically active on a regular basis still show increases in muscle strength, size, and flexibility even into their 90s.

Film action hero Sylvester Stallone is an excellent well-known example of a man who at age 67 is more active and better physically fit than most Americans in their 30s. At age 70, the legendary Jack Lalanne still performed feats in public such as swimming one full mile in open water while towing 60–70 rowboats behind him.

Lesser known, but just as impressive, are guys like Cliff Eggink, who at the age of 70 was still participating in triathlon contests, which included over 2 miles of swimming, 100 miles of bike riding, and 26 miles of marathon course running. There are now approximately 200,000 Americans over the age of 40 officially registered and participating in

Masters sporting events that include marathons, distance swimming, and triathlons.

Your initial reaction may be to dismiss these examples as rare exceptions and freaks of nature. But such is not the case. These people were not all blessed with perfect genetics that magically made them different from you or anybody else. The only difference between most of them and today's vision of the statistical norm is the choices they make and the way they live their lives.

Realistically, nobody is going to try to claim a perfectly fit person at age 65 is going to be in better condition than a trained athlete at age 23. Such a claim would be foolish and misleading.

But, it has been demonstrated by numerous studies that a combination of weight resistance training, cardiovascular exercise, and an intelligent daily diet routine can slow the aging process and even reverse many of the negative effects brought about by years of self-neglect. Under these conditions, it is not uncommon to see individuals in their 60s and even older who can leave many younger people in the dust.

These encouraging words are supported by research conducted by Dr. Vonda Wright and published in the March 2008 edition of the *American Journal of Sports Medicine*. In this study, Dr. Wright analyzed the conditioning and performance of senior athletes aged 50 to 85.

It was observed that overall race times and other measurements of physical performance demonstrated only a small, slow, and steady decline until age 75. Between the years of 50 and 75, these athlete's race times became slower by less than 2% per year.

Dr. Wright has spent many years studying the effects of aging on athletes and physical performance during each step of the aging process. After many years of study and repeated statistical results, there seems to be some conclusions that can be drawn from her findings:

- Until age 75, there does not appear to be any major natural decline in a human system that has been well maintained, fed properly, and exercised intelligently.

- The natural decline in human performance and conditioning from ages 30 to 50 is only that resulting from the earliest stages of the aging process from our ultimate physical peaks.

- The natural rate of performance decline between the ages of 50 to 75 equates to less than 2% per year.

- Age 75 appears to be the point where the human biological system is designed by nature to begin a quicker rate of performance and function loss.

To be certain, there are people well into their 90s who are still very active and could put an average 50-year-old to shame, but we are talking statistical norms here. It seems nature did not intend for the human body to experience any major loss of performance or independence prior to the age of 75. It can be argued that any major decline in physical capability before this age is probably due to disease, injury, genetics, or unhealthy lifestyle choices.

If we are fortunate enough to avoid serious injury, extremely bad genetics, or disease, then a lifestyle consisting of a balanced diet and structured exercise routine should allow the majority of us to remain active, energetic, and independent until age 75.

Bottom line—age 75 seems to be the point where nature really intended the human machine to begin slowing down.

We Are Not Twenty Anymore—But What Does That Really Mean?

When we are young, our bodies are able to tolerate a fair degree of abuse and neglect. Late night parties, bad eating habits, burning the candle at both ends, and getting by on 3–4 hours of sleep for weeks at a time—it seems this is a common way for many people to spend at least some portion of their youth.

Back then, all it took was a few days of returning to better habits and you felt 100% again. Chances are, you gave much less concern to your health 20+ years ago, but still managed to look and feel pretty good anyway.

Now, let us fast forward to this morning. If you are like most people over 40, you awoke with some aches and pains. Perhaps it was your lower back, perhaps you felt and even heard clicking and popping in your shoulders. When you took your first steps, was there pain in your heels or the soles of your feet? Perhaps you even bear the reminders of surgical procedures.

Congratulations, you are not twenty any more. These aches and pains are merit badges of courage earned and accumulated over a lifetime of experiences and activities.

But there are more important things to consider than only a variety of aches and pains. Starting at around age 30, a number of biological factors begin to occur in our bodies. These subtle changes signal the beginning of a gradual decline of our abilities that we experience over the remainder of our lives.

At first, the thought of slowing metabolism, lost muscle mass, increased fat, reduced flexibility, shortness of breath, aching joints, less energy, sexual dysfunction, and brittle bones may invoke a slight feeling of despair.

Fear not. Being over 40, you have a big advantage over the 20-year-old version of yourself: Wisdom and Experience. How many times have you heard the phrase, *If I only knew then what I know now?* Chances are you have said this to yourself many times over the years.

It is true. Many times we don't learn the right way to do things until later in life. Perhaps we did not have the patience or self-discipline when we were younger. Maybe we thought we knew all the answers. Maybe we were lucky and things worked out OK, not because of what we did, but despite what we may have done. Whatever the reason, it is not uncommon to see people sometimes excel at a certain activity after the age of 40.

What does this mean in regards to our discussion of 40 no longer necessarily being the point where we are doomed to rapidly fall apart? It means if we have an understanding of what exactly is happening inside our bodies as we age, we can make intelligent changes to partially neutralize those effects and improve our overall level of fitness and performance. These changes can make us look and feel much younger than the majority of people our same age in the general population.

Let's take a look at what happens as we pass the normal physiological peak of age 30 and how the program detailed later in this book can help you to slow and minimize these effects.

Muscle Fiber and Your Metabolism

The human body reaches a peak of muscle conditioning around the age of 30. Assuming no significant changes to daily activity levels, we lose 0.5–1.0% of muscle tissue each year after that. This means the average 50-year-old, having made no adjustments to their lifestyle during this time, may see as much as 10–20% less muscle size and strength.

Skeletal muscle is not just important for defining the shape of our bodies and how we fill out our clothing, it is also directly tied to the way our body uses calories.

Your body has something called the Basal Metabolic Rate (BMR). Essentially BMR is the amount of energy or calories your body needs when at rest to perform vital survival functions such as digesting food, inflating lungs, beating the heart, allowing your brain to function, etc. This BMR can be thought of as the number of calories your body requires to function when it is sitting at idle.

Your BMR is closely tied to the amount of lean muscle mass your body possesses. The reason for this correlation is because your skeletal muscles are essentially your body's engine. Just as with an automobile, the larger the engine the more fuel it will consume when sitting at idle as compared to a smaller engine.

If, for example, between the ages of 30 and 50, a sedentary person experiences an average 20% of muscle loss, yet fails to either increase their activity levels OR reduce calorie consumption, they will gain weight. It is simple mathematics. To compound this problem, since most people continue to eat the same way at 50 as they may have eaten at age 20, they are prone to gain extra fat more quickly as they lose muscle mass.

A vicious cycle is created. The loss of skeletal muscle mass causes the BMR rate to lower. This lowered Basal Metabolic Rate combines with the natural slowing of the metabolism to decrease the body's daily calorie requirements. If you continue to eat the same amount and types of food as you did 30 years earlier when you had both a faster natural metabolism and more muscle mass, the result is excess weight gain. Carrying extra weight, a person feels more tired and sluggish and finds it harder to get involved in any form of physical activity.

As the amount of physical activity declines yet again, there is a further decrease in stimulation to grow or maintain skeletal muscle and the metabolic rate drops even further. This cycle continues again and again with an ever-increasing amount of excess fat and body weight being accumulated. So how do we overcome this problem?

Here is the first of many important principles that are useful to remember and adhere to. You will find them highlighted throughout this book.

✦ Important Principle ✦

Your Body's Metabolic Rate is Largely Determined By Skeletal Muscle Mass. If You Allow Muscles to Atrophy With Age, Your Metabolic Rate Will Drop and Gaining Fat Will Become Easier.

Without question, studies too numerous to count have shown regular weight resistance training to be the solution to greatly reducing the typical rate of muscle loss seen by the average sedentary citizen.

When we talk about weight resistance training, we are not referring to the image that may first pop into your mind—that of an Olympic power lifter trying to hoist 400 pounds over his head in a massive, gut-busting effort. Weight resistance training as defined here is a program of exercises designed to work all the major muscle groups of the body with enough effort so as to stimulate the continued regeneration and growth of muscle fibers.

This type of program requires the individual to exert enough effort such that they are pushing the muscles to work right up to the point of failure. This "failure" is the point where the muscle has fatigued and can no longer continue that movement against the current resistance without a rest. Since the body is highly adaptive to external stimulus, a regular routine that forces the muscle to confront a workload that is slightly beyond its current abilities triggers the regeneration and growth we need to prevent the fading away of our natural lean muscle mass.

As discussed earlier in this chapter, recent research has shown that weight resistance training is beneficial at all stages of our life. Intuitively this makes sense if you think about it. After all, we require muscles to walk, carry, and move throughout our entire lives. If the muscles are indeed the engine that allows our body to move around in our world, it makes sense that we would like that engine to be running as strongly as possible.

Don't think you are too old to benefit. In a recent study headed by Wayne L. Westcott, PhD, working with nursing home patients in Massachusetts, the benefits of weight resistance training were clearly demonstrated. The results of this study conformed with and supported similar studies performed in recent years.

The patients averaged 88.5 years of age. They underwent a 14-week strength training program that incorporated many of the principles you will learn in this book. At the end of this study, the patients experienced an overall weight gain of 1 pound, with a body fat composition decrease of 2%. This increase in weight with simultaneous body fat reduction shows an impressive increase in muscle tissue.

Perhaps even more important than the measured changes in muscle to fat ratio was the improvement in functional strength. On the basic leg press and triceps press used to evaluate leg and arm strength, the patients experienced a 47-pound increase in the amount of weight they could lift with their legs, and a 15-pound increase in the amount of weight they could press with their arms. Compared to their abilities at the start of the study, this equates to an 81% and 39% improvement in the amount of weight that could be lifted using the legs and arms respectively.

Keep in mind, these were people living in a nursing home, averaging almost 89 years of age, that participated in only 14 weeks of the type of weight resistance program we are discussing in this book. Weight resistance training will help maintain your skeletal muscle mass, which in turn will keep you stronger, more mobile, and assist in preventing excess weight gain.

Calcium Depletion and Loss of Bone Density

A house is only as strong as its frame. For our bodies, the framework, upon which all our muscles, tendons, and organs are attached, is the skeleton. The human skeleton is composed of over 206 bones.

Bone tissue is a combination of a dense outer cortex with a sponge-like inner matrix which has the dynamic ability to adapt and change shape depending on the stresses placed upon it. If one takes a moment to think how well broken bones heal after an accident, this technical fact is made even more impressive.

 After peaking around the age of 30, there is a general decline in bone density. The inner matrix of the bones becomes less efficient at reutilizing calcium and other minerals to rebuild and repair the structure network that gives bones their strength.

Women are particularly more susceptible to, and impacted by, bone loss due to hormonal influences on calcium retention. In fact, after the age of 40 women tend to lose bone density at twice the rate of men. After menopause, the rate of bone loss accelerates once again. It is for this reason we see most advertisements for calcium supplements and warnings about osteoporosis aimed at women.

While women are particularly more susceptible and impacted by bone loss and calcium depletion, it is a concern for everyone as we age. We have all seen the trademark signs of serious bone loss and osteoporosis. These signs include shortened height in the aged, stooped posture, and broken hips. These are the most commonly recognized symptoms that indicate an advanced degree of bone loss.

Once again our new friend, weight resistance training, can help us guard against this common effect of aging. Combined with calcium and vitamin D3 supplementation, progressive weight training stimulates the bone tissue to increase its regeneration activity.

Why is this? It seems as with the case of muscle fiber, the bones also obey the commonly heard phrase "use it or lose it." The human body is very adaptive to long-term continuous and progressive stimulus. If you continue to impose a force on your body that is greater than what it would experience in an otherwise sedentary environment, it will increase the size and strength of your muscles and density of the bones to be better able to deal with the new workload. Weight resistance training, combined with a proper dietary intake of calcium and vitamin D, will help ward off osteoporosis and keep your bones strong for many more years as compared to a sedentary individual.

Your Heart and Pumping Capacity

People are always amazed at the design and performance of the human heart. Over a typical lifetime, the heart will beat over 3 billion times without ever taking a full rest *(that's 100,000 times per day)*. Unlike all other muscles in the body, it is one organ that works non-stop from the time we are born until the day we die.

Everyday the amazing heart is required to pump the equivalent of 1,800 gallons of blood through 60,000 miles of combined blood vessels. In a healthy person, the heart is happy to perform this daily duty reliably and with no protest. But with age, the heart is often forced to work harder. Interestingly enough, it does not appear that the natural aging of the heart is its main cause of decline.

The primary cause for changes in the heart appears to be clogged and hardened arteries that place an increasingly harder demand on the pumping effort over time.

Hardening of the arteries is most commonly caused when the blood vessels become narrowed due to fat and cholesterol becoming deposited on the inside walls of the arteries. These deposits can harden over time via fibrous tissue formation and calcification. If you live in an older house or have a hard water supply you have probably seen a perfect visual example of what happens to blood vessels as they go through this process.

A simple experiment will help you appreciate your heart a little more. Purse your lips and blow. This should be easy and effortless.

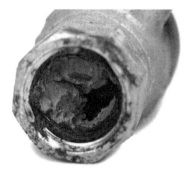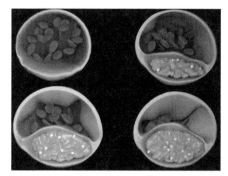

(Photo 2.1) Old plumbing and scale formation is a perfect analogy to aged blood vessels.

Now do the same thing but place your finger over your lips as though you are telling somebody to be quiet. Try to exhale the same amount of air. What happens? You will feel your cheeks expand with back pressure. There will be a natural tendency to try to blow a little harder to expel the air at the same speed.

If you imagine this air is blood and your cheeks are the muscle walls of your heart, you can better appreciate how hardened arteries and restricted flow volume due to arteriosclerosis greatly increases the workload on your heart. You can better understand how even a small increase in physical effort might place a demand on the heart that it can't compensate for.

A heart attack may be the final result. Looking at statistics derived from medical study, the following changes are normally seen with an aging heart:

- The left ventricle wall enlarges to compensate for increased resistance due to narrowed arteries. This results in a harder, more forceful pumping heart at the expense of increased blood pressure.

- For reasons not yet understood, the heart is slower to react to chemical messages from the brain as the years pass by. This means the heart does not rapidly adjust to changes in workload as it did when younger. The result is a decrease in energy intensity and activity endurance exhibited by a shortness of breath. Since the heart is not circulating oxygen-rich blood fast enough to meet the needs of the more active body, the lungs begin gasping for more air to try to compensate by increasing the amount of oxygen available to the system.

- With age, our resting heart rate slows. In order to compensate, the heart pumps more blood with each individual beat, resulting in an increased diastolic pressure. Diastolic pressure is the bottom number in your blood pressure reading. It represents the resting pressure of the blood in your arteries in the pause between beats. As you may already know, a high diastolic pressure is of concern since it indicates the heart and blood vessels never get a break and are always under a higher than normal degree of pressure. Think of a garden hose left laying in the yard with the main water valve left open. The constant pressure on the hose will cause it to rupture much earlier than a hose which is emptied and relieved of all pressure after use.

- Due to the increase in diastolic blood pressure, the heart stretches larger with each beat. While this gives a stronger pump and contraction to move the excess blood volume, the greater diastolic pressure prevents the heart from squeezing as tightly as it did when younger.

- The heart of a healthy person at age 70 has 30% fewer cells than that of a healthy 20-year-old. When heart cells die, the remaining cells stretch and grow to fill the void so as to maintain integrity. This results in an older person's heart cells being as much as 40% larger than that of a younger person.

Some quick statistics to put all this heart information into perspective :

- 40% of deaths between the ages of 65–74 are caused by heart disease.

- 60% of deaths after the age of 80 are the result of heart disease.

- Between the ages of 20 and 80, there is a 50% decline in the body's capacity for vigorous activity.

- Between the ages of 20 and 80, the heart's maximum heart rate drops from approximately 190bpm down to 145bpm.

- At age 20, the heart can increase output up to 4 times its resting capacity. By age 80, this ramp up ability is limited to double capacity.

The combination of healthy diet and exercise as described in this book can drastically reduce the typical rate at which arteries become blocked and hardened.

Your Lungs and Oxygen Exchange Capability

When was the last time you walked up a set of steps or a steep hill and were shocked by how quickly you became short of breath? For those people living an extensively sedentary lifestyle, sometimes the simple act of walking to the mailbox at the curb, or walking down the stairs to their basement, can seem like a tiring effort that leaves them panting for air.

As you may have guessed, this is NOT a normal condition of fitness for any person under the age of 75. The heart may be responsible for supplying oxygenated blood to your muscles, organs, and other tissues so they may perform their essential functions, but it is the lungs which must first bring that oxygen from the outside world into your body.

The lungs have two primary functions. First, they acquire oxygen from the air, which is required for life. Secondly, they remove carbon dioxide from the body. Carbon dioxide is a major byproduct of many of the chemical reactions that occur in our bodies as we sustain life. When we breathe, the oxygen in the air we inhale attaches itself to red blood cells. This oxygenated blood is circulated by the heart to all the waiting tissues in our bodies.

As we pass the age of 30, more energy and effort is required to breathe. One reason for this increased effort is due to a steady decline in our maximum breathing capacity. Sometimes called "vital capacity," this maximum amount of air that our lungs are able to hold decreases as much as 40% by the time we reach the age of 75.

Along with this decrease in vital capacity, the lungs lose a degree of elasticity, which makes full expansion more difficult. Additionally, a steady decline in capillaries and a diminished ability of oxygen exchange inside the lungs decreases the efficiency at which oxygen and carbon dioxide are managed inside the lungs.

The maximum force you can generate when inhaling and exhaling also decreases with age, as the diaphragm and muscles between the ribs become weaker. The chest cavity is then less able to stretch during inhalation and exhalation, causing the pattern of breathing to alter slightly as compensation for this decreased ability to expand the chest. With this loss of efficiency, each breath we take is less effective at expelling carbon dioxide and absorbing oxygen.

With less total lung capacity and lowered oxygen/carbon dioxide exchange efficiency available in each individual breath, the body resorts to increasing the number of breathes to try to compensate for the oxygen debt. When we physically exert ourselves beyond our normal baseline level of activity, the sensation of panting and gasping for breath is usually the result. This sensation is essentially our lung's attempt to intake a larger volume of air to get the oxygen our body needs.

It goes without saying that smoking is an absolute no-no for keeping the lungs in healthy shape. I confess I have never understood the concept or fascination with smoking. The habit itself has always seemed bizarre to me.

I often question the mentality of that first human who thought it would be a good idea to dry leaves, crush them up, set them on fire, and intentionally inhale the smoke into his body. How did he ever think that was a good idea? When you step back from the familiarity of the habit and look at it as an outside observer seeing it for the first time, you must admit there is little logic to the practice of smoking.

The good news is that weight training and cardiovascular exercise go a long way towards maintaining peak performance of the lungs. As we will see later in the chapter dealing with exercise, 30 minutes of cardiovascular training three times per week combined with weight training allows the lungs to retain a large degree of their elasticity and expansion capacity as we age. This type of regimen also keeps the oxygen/carbon dioxide exchange capacity of the lungs functioning closer to their younger peak levels.

Endurance and Energy

One of the most common complaints of getting older is the feeling that we simply don't have the energy to do anything anymore. I imagine you have heard people make the comment, "I know I should exercise, but I'm too tired from normal daily activities to think about exercising. All I want to do is lie down on the couch and watch TV."

To be certain, we all feel like this from time to time. Perhaps it has been an especially tough week at work. Maybe there are some family emergencies weighing on your mind and causing extra fatigue. We all have times when we need to take a detour from our normal routine and let our inner batteries recharge. But for some people, this feeling of being tired all the time is a constant way of life. They almost never feel energetic and alive.

As discussed earlier, most modern research into human physiology seems to indicate that in the absence of any major illness or injury, the human machine is not designed by nature to show a dramatic decline in capability until we pass our mid 70s. I have an interesting story to demonstrate this fact.

Several years ago my wife and I took a lengthy tour of Asia. One day of sightseeing was spent visiting the Great Wall of China. As it happens, there were two ways for visitors to ascend the Great Wall. One path led up a more gradual and gentle slope to view the mountains and vistas. Another path was for the more adventurous as it required walking up a steeper section of the Wall to an even higher elevation.

On the drive from our hotel to the Great Wall, our tour guide told us to be on the lookout for an elderly couple who had become local legends in recent years. This elderly Chinese couple was in their 90s and had been married since they were in their 20s. They lived in a nearby village and had a relatively simple life of farming. They also hand-crafted textiles that were sold in local markets. The tour guide explained that this couple had made a habit of walking together up the steeper section of the Wall every day of their lives for the past 70 years.

We arrived at the visitor center mid-morning and were instantly besieged by locals trying to sell all manner of souvenirs, shirts, books, and local handicrafts. My wife and I chose to join the tourists brave enough to tackle the steeper path up the Great Wall. We hoped to enjoy the magnificent views that had been promised to those willing to accept the challenge of this more rigorous trek.

I must admit the steeper route up the Great Wall of China felt at times very much like walking on a stair-climber machine, or a treadmill with the incline at full elevation. Regardless of age, everybody in the tour group took rest stops at various times to catch their breath on the way to the zenith. However, there were at least two people who climbed the same path that day without ever stopping to take a rest of any kind.

When we were approximately half way to our destination, I heard small, rapid footsteps on the stone walkway behind me. About this same time, I began to hear cameras clicking and the murmur of awed voices in English, German, French, Italian, and several other languages belonging to the patrons of other tour groups who were with us that day. I turned to see a man and woman, both dressed in traditional black Chinese garb. They were small in stature, as are most Chinese who have lived a life untouched by the modern dietary influences of the West. Like two little marching machines, they were walking hand in hand up this steep slope of the Great Wall at a pace that left all us tourists in the dust.

While the majority of tourists (aged 25–65) stood gasping for breath, this 92-year-old couple whisked by without making any sound outside the regular pacing of their footsteps. They simply walked past the crowd with a small nod and smile and continued on their way.

That day was a real eye-opener for me. Yes, we have been told forever how exercise and regular activity is essential for health and longevity. The truth is, most people know this is good advice, but they still maintain reservations, thinking it is a bunch of hype and pep-talk.

In our hearts, we know this is time-proven wisdom and not simply motivational speaking. In fact, we have all seen firsthand a perfect demonstration of how rapidly the body can decline as a result of disuse.

Have you or any friends ever had a broken arm? Remember what that arm looked like when it was removed from the cast weeks later? After only 3–5 weeks of inactivity, that arm was smaller in size, weak, stiff, and lacked coordination of movement.

While an arm in a cast may be an extreme example of inactivity's effect on the body, it is still very relevant. The human body thrives on activity. It is this same reason so many people can often be heard making the comment, "I didn't feel like going to the gym today, but I am glad I went. I feel much better now."

Years ago, we worked on farms. We ate what we grew, worked hard all day long, and had no problem getting a good night's sleep. Today, most people eat too much junk from fast food restaurants, sit behind a desk during the day, and lay on a couch watching TV at night. Then they need prescription medications to help them go to sleep. Technology has improved in amazing ways, but other aspects of our society and health have actually taken a step backwards and worsened.

In the preceding section, we emphasized how the right combination of diet, weight resistance training, and cardiovascular conditioning can benefit us and slow the typical declines we see in muscle, heart, artery, lungs, and bone health.

When all these body organs are working synergistically at a high level of performance, the natural result is increased energy, stamina, and endurance. By contrast, if a person is carrying an extra 50 pounds of dead weight on them in the form of fat, never allowing his heart and lungs to condition themselves to a higher level of performance, and is clogging his blood vessels with fatty deposits—then of course there is going to be a notable decline in energy levels.

One might consider the difference between two automobiles to serve as a suitable analogy. The first car has been well-maintained with regular oil changes and tune-ups. It has been washed and waxed every few months and has regular changes of brake fluid, transmission fluid, etc.

Even though this vehicle is well past 130,000 miles, it still runs smoothly and reliably. There is a good chance this car could reach and surpass 300,000 miles if well-maintained in this fashion.

The second car has basically been driven with no thought to regular maintenance. Only when the vehicle totally breaks down and quits running does it receive any kind of care or service. The oil gets changed every 20,000 miles (maybe). It has never had a change of spark plugs, or a new air cleaner in ten years. The gas still pumps (or seeps) through the same fuel filter that came with the car when it was new (or last broke down and required emergency service). The only water this car has ever seen is from rain, and nobody has ever thought to check the brake fluid, transmission fluid, or any other vital system.

Chances are this car does not run very well and has broken down a few times, leaving the driver stranded. Most likely, this second auto will not survive long enough to see 200,000 miles.

Looking good is certainly nice. But feeling good is even better. As we pass the peak years of 30–40, we can't rely on youth to compensate and protect us from the way we treat ourselves. With the passing of years, a wise combination of diet, supplementation, and exercise can help maintain a more youthful level of energy. You CAN have much more endurance and energy than is often seen and accepted in middle age and older.

Flexibility and Mobility

Okay—time for a simple test.

Don't attempt this if you knowingly have any serious back or joint problems and are under a doctor's supervision restricting range of motion or flexibility. For everybody else, here we go:

1. Stand up with your legs straight. Do not bend your knees.
2. Now slowly bend forward at the waist *(keep those knees straight)*.
3. Now touch the floor with the palms of your hands *(your hands should be just in front of your toes – see Photo 2.2)*.

Only those people with exceptionally long legs or short arms should have a problem with this flexibility test if they are otherwise in good shape. This flexibility test has been popular for many years in fitness and yoga circles.

Interestingly enough, 60 years ago it was reported that almost 70% of people could successfully perform this test. Today, it seems only 35% of the general population can exhibit this level of flexibility.

What has changed? There are several factors that help explain why the average person in today's society has a harder time performing this

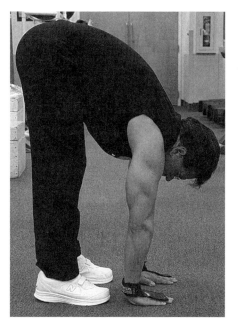

(Photo 2.2) Basic Flexibility Test. Keeping knees straight, touch the palms of your hands to the floor.

flexibility test as compared to our predecessors.

• 30% of Americans today are now considered obese. Excess fat stored around the middle physically limits the ability to bend at the waist.

• A sedentary lifestyle does not allow the muscles, tendons, and ligaments to regularly work through a full range of motion. This results in a shortening and stiffening of these tissues, leading to a smaller degree of mobility.

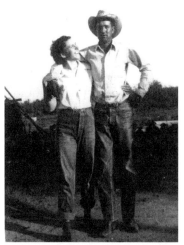
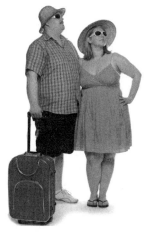

(Photo 2.3) The body composition of the "average" person has changed over the past 60 years.

Assuming we all want to be able to see our own toes and tie our own shoelaces as we grow older, let's take a closer look at the four largest factors that effect our flexibility.

Excess Weight

The first factor that limits flexibility is extra body fat. The simple presence of extra fat around the joints introduces a physical obstruction that limits the ability for that portion of the body to move through a full length of travel.

Imagine a door on a hinge. That door can easily and fully swing open and closed. The hinge of a door closely resembles the structural mechanics of your own knee, elbow, and to some degree, the forward bending motion of the waist.

Now place a pillow or other object near that door's hinge. The range of travel will be limited as you try to swing the door. At some point, if you continue to try to force the door open against the resistance, you may even break the hinges. This is equivalent to the extra stress potentially imposed on the joints in our body if enough excess body fat is allowed to accumulate around them.

Years ago, a popular misconception was that bodybuilders and other athletes with large muscular structure were muscle-bound and clumsy. The fact is that even with muscular development considerably larger than the average person, most athletes and bodybuilders are still able to perform the flexibility test described at the beginning of this section.

How is this possible? If you look closely at a well-developed muscular physique, you will observe the main mass of the muscle is in the middle of the tissue. We call this the muscle belly. The origin and insertion points for those muscles are normally tapered near the joints. This is a much different scenario than exists with excess body fat, which tends to deposit itself pretty much everyplace you don't want it.

As a result, the flexing of a muscle does not interfere with the movement of a joint in the same way as "lifeless" fat does. There is a common saying in sports circles —*You can't flex fat.*

Certainly there are a small percentage of professional bodybuilders at the rare extreme levels of the sport who have an almost freakish level of muscular hypertrophy. These people also take large dosages of steroids and growth hormone and demonstrate a level of muscular growth that is not attainable to the normal person. At this size, certainly some limited mobility can become an issue simply as a result of the extreme body mass, but in our discussions here we are looking at the normal person or athlete and not that rare 0.25% of extreme bodybuilders.

Muscle Tissue Changes

We spoke earlier about how lean muscle mass is directly tied to metabolism and the ability to avoid gaining excess weight as we age.

With time, muscles tend to become stiffer due to a decreased ability to hold water, loss of cells, and changes in the way the fibers cross link during contraction. Looking a little deeper, we learn muscles are actually composed of two types of fiber:

Type I (Slow Twitch Fibers) – These muscle fibers are not capable of strong, explosive power, but they excel at providing endurance and long-duration lower-intensity movement.

Type II (Fast Twitch Fibers) – These muscle fibers provide you with power and strength. While they do not have a high level of endurance, they provide explosive power to lift heavy objects, jump up from a chair quickly in an emergency, or throw a hard punch to defend yourself in a fight.

We all have approximately a 50/50 ratio of these fibers in our muscles. The small genetic variances each of us has in this ratio of fibers helps explain why we have more natural ability at certain physical activities.

For example, one person with a higher ratio of Type I (slow twitch endurance fibers) may find it easier to run long distance marathons or swim the English Channel. By comparison, another person with a higher ratio of Type II (fast twitch power fibers) may find sprinting or power lifting comes more naturally to them.

As we age, we lose both types of muscle fiber—but NOT at the same rate. Research has shown that as we age, Type II (fast twitch power fibers) atrophy at almost twice the speed of Type I (slow twitch endurance fibers). This may help explain why an average healthy 70-year-old has little problem taking long walks or spending a full day sightseeing at an amusement park. But this same individual might find it more difficult to turn a mattress, or quickly jump up from a chair when the phone rings. As the research indicates, this person still has a higher percentage of Type I fibers which give them endurance, but they have lost substantially more Type II fibers which provides for power, strength, and faster movements.

Later, when we start discussing the exact exercise routine you will be performing three times per week, we will talk more about this difference in muscle fiber composition and how to stimulate their growth. But for now, we introduce this concept since it has been determined that Type II fibers also seem to have the wider range of flexibility as required by their ability to generate quick and explosive power. The important thing to remember now is we must regularly exercise these muscle fibers with some form of resistance training that follows a full and natural range of motion. This practice will prevent the loss of flexibility that would otherwise occur from passive, sedentary aging.

Tendons & Ligaments

People sometimes confuse tendons and ligaments. To help clarify the difference between the two structures, some short definitions are in order:

Tendon – a tough band of tissue that connects muscles to bone.

Ligament – fibrous tissue that connects bones to other bones.

As we age, both of these tissues lose elasticity and flexibility for a variety of reasons similar to what is seen in muscle aging. Water content decreases, cellular healing falters, injuries and micro-tears accumulate over a lifetime of use.

Most readers will be familiar with the common ailment of tendonitis or specifically tennis elbow. This painful condition results from excessive repetition of the same motion against an opposing force (in this case hitting a tennis ball thousands of times per week). This relentless pressure on the forearm creates small micro-tears and inflammation at the junction of the muscles and tendon. Usually in the case of tennis elbow, this is felt on the lateral (outside) point of the elbow and can extend over the top of the forearm.

When a structure such as a tendon is injured, the immune system is stimulated to try to repair the injured area. Since both ligaments and tendons have limited blood supplies, slow and/or incomplete healing is common after these types of injuries. This slow healing often results in decreased strength of the area.

The ligaments and tendons are normally tight, strong bands of fibrous or connective tissue, but injury causes them to become relaxed and weak. An injured ligament or tendon then becomes a source of chronic pain and weakness that can last for weeks or months. All of this is one of the reasons most professional athletes fear major injuries to tendons and ligaments above almost all else.

As anybody who has suffered tendonitis knows, one of the most commonly prescribed therapies for recovery besides medication is stretching. This is because continued misuse of these tendons in the same manner over time will lead to a tightening of the fibers. Tightened fibers unable to stretch throughout their normal range are more prone to injury.

Cartilage

People suffering with lower back problems may already know more than they care to about cartilage deterioration.

Cartilage is the flexible connective tissue found in many areas of our bodies, including the joints between bones, the rib cage, the ear, the nose, and especially intervertebral discs. This type of tissue is not as hard and rigid as bone, but it is stiffer and less flexible than muscle. Unlike other connective tissue in the body, cartilage has no blood supply and has limited healing ability. For this reason, cartilage heals and repairs much more slowly than tendons and ligaments.

Osteoarthritis, rheumatoid arthritis, and gout are all ailments we potentially face as we age. Degeneration or destruction of cartilage is the major force behind these three conditions.

To be more specific:

Osteoarthritis
This condition (also known as degenerative arthritis) is a painful and increasingly debilitating disease. Eventually, the cartilage residing on the end of the bones is completely lost. This results from either damage or inflammatory degeneration. Eventually the result is bone rubbing against bone. Swelling, inflammation, and pain are common. The joint pain can render a person unable to perform tasks such as common movement, lifting, and even simple walking. Under extreme conditions, treatment may involve joint replacement surgery.

Rheumatoid arthritis

This is a chronic system-wide inflammatory autoimmune disease. Rheumatoid arthritis targets synovial joints. Synovial joints are the most common and movable joints in the body. The process of rheumatoid arthritis leads to the destruction of cartilage and rigidity of the joint and may affect other areas of the body. Unlike osteoarthritis, which occurs primarily in later years, rheumatoid arthritis can affect people of almost any age.

Gout (inflammatory arthritis)

This is a condition caused by elevated levels of uric acid in the blood. The uric acid crystallizes, and the crystals deposit in joints, tendons, and surrounding tissues. Gout is characterized by the frequent reoccurrence of acute inflammatory arthritis, producing a red, tender, and painful swelling of the joint. If gout is not managed through medications, supplementation, and lifestyle changes, the repeated bouts of inflammation can cause permanent damage to cartilage.

The routines described later in this book include morning wake-up stretching moves, along with exercises designed to provide a full range of motion for all major muscle groups.

Exercising regularly with a full range of motion helps to keep your connective tissue as healthy as possible. Combined with a healthy diet and selected supplementation, we can do much to maintain youthful flexibility and mobility well into our later years.

Sexual Function

Sex and aging is a delicate subject many people are not comfortable talking about. However, it is a part of the human experience, and should not be avoided in a discussion of how we change past the age of 40.

The most obvious transition point for women comes at menopause. During menopause, decreased estrogen levels bring about physical and emotional changes that can affect not only the biological aspects of sexual activity but also mental attitude and self-perception.

For women, some of the effects introduced by aging include:

- Loss of elasticity and a thinning of the vaginal tissue.

- Decrease in the amount of lubrication.

- Decrease in the size of clitoral and labial tissues, although clitoral sensitivity remains the same.

- Decrease in the size of the cervix, uterus, and ovaries.

- The anticipation and build up to orgasm often decreases while climax itself may also be less intense.

- Sexual desire may be reduced due to a combination of these biological changes, combined with self image issues dealing with excess weight or physical appearance.

A large part of sex is feeling sexy. Women who exercise typically have an improved body image over those who do not exercise. Feeling better about their bodies usually leads to a more positive attitude towards sex. A study conducted a few years ago revealed that 60% of women who exercised three times weekly rated their own sexual desirability as above average.

For men, some of the effects introduced by aging include:

- Erections may not be as hard or may be totally absent in the case of impotence.

- Erections take longer to occur while the recovery time for subsequent erections may increase to as long as 12 to 24 hours.

- Fewer sperm are produced.

- The force of ejaculation decreases.

- As with women, sexual desire may be reduced due to a combination of biological changes, combined with self image issues resulting from excess weight or physical appearance.

Many of the problems men face with aging are the result of declining testosterone levels. As a man ages his testosterone level decreases. Typically this decrease in testosterone becomes evident when a man is in his 40s. The first symptom of lowered testosterone may be a tougher time building muscle while fat deposits itself more easily around the midsection. Often levels do not drop low enough to cause sexual problems until the age of 55–60.

Testosterone is not the only factor which can cause sexual function problems in men. As Steven Lamm, MD, at the New York University School of Medicine states, "the harder the erection the healthier the man." What Doctor Lamm is referring to in his bold and slightly racy statement is the recently discovered correlation between the strength of male erections and the associated condition of the overall cardiovascular system. The condition of the heart and arteries affect how blood flows in the body. When the arteries become narrower and harder, blood does not flow as freely. This reduced blood flow can be troublesome for men trying to achieve an erection since erections are highly dependent upon the ability of blood to fill the penis.

Exercise keeps the heart and arteries healthy, thus reducing the risk of erectile dysfunction. Researchers conducting a study of men over the age of 50 found that those who were physically active reported better erections and a 30% lower incidence of impotence as compared to men who were inactive.

Television advertisements for medications such as Viagra have become as prevalent today as commercials for laundry detergent. Based on our discussion above, it might come as no surprise that the original intended use for Sildenafil Citrate (Viagra) was for the treatment of cardiovascular conditions and blood pressure. However, one of the unexpected side effects of the drug was its ability to attain and maintain an erection—causing the medication to jokingly be called the "Pfizer Riser." The rest, one might say, is history—a product making more money from an unexpected side effect than from its original intended purpose.

The lesson to be learned here is that controlling high blood pressure and other cardiovascular diseases through lifestyle changes, diet, and exercise can improve sexual performance and possibly delay or prevent the need for male enhancement medications. In both men and women, the combined physical and mental benefits of weight control, exercise, and diet go a long way to ensure a sexually active relationship well into your later years.

Mood Enhancement & Offsetting Depression

Over 19 million people in the United States and an estimated 121 million worldwide suffer some degree of constant anxiety or outright depression. Traditionally the treatment for anxiety and depression has been a combination of psychological counseling and the use of various classes of antidepressant medications.

While there is no doubt that a percentage of severe depression cases and anxiety require extensive use of therapy and medications, an increasing number of recent studies indicate we are overprescribing patients when other treatments may be just as effective and possibly more desirable.

A number of university and clinical studies have shown a combination of exercise, dietary changes, and supplementation to be just as effective as drugs in a large number of patients suffering from depression. Also of interest is the fact that the benefits in many cases appear to be longer lasting.

The Effect of Exercise on Depression Symptoms
Following a study that demonstrated that 30 minutes of brisk exercise three times a week is just as effective as drug treatment in relieving the

symptoms of major depression over the short term, Duke University researchers took their research further to show that continued exercise greatly reduces the chances of depression returning.

The original Duke study focused on 156 older patients diagnosed with major depression, who after 16 weeks of routine exercise showed statistically significant improvement relative to those who took anti-depression medications, or those who took the medication and exercised.

The newer study, which followed the same participants for an additional six months, found those patients who continued to exercise after completing the initial trial were less likely to see their depression symptoms return than the other patients. Only 8% of patients in the exercise group had their depression return, while 38% of the drug-only group and 31% of the exercise-plus-drug group relapsed.

Duke psychologist James Blumenthal, who published the results of the study in the October 2000 issue of the journal *Psychosomatic Medicine* remarked, "The important conclusion is that the effectiveness of exercise seems to persist over time, and that patients who respond well to exercise and maintain their exercise have a much smaller risk of relapsing."

Blumenthal goes on to explain, "We found that there was an inverse relationship between exercise and the risk of relapsing. The more one exercised, the less likely one would see their depressive symptoms return. For each 50-minute increment of exercise, there was an associated 50% reduction in relapse. Findings from these studies indicate that a modest exercise program is an effective and robust treatment for patients with major depression, and if these motivated patients continue with their exercise, they have a much better chance of not seeing their depression return."

One unexpected observation from the study was the fact that the group of patients who took the medication and exercised did not respond as well as those who only exercised. Blumenthal comments, "We had assumed that exercise and medication together would have had an additive effect, but this turned out not to be the case. While we don't know the reasons for this, some of the participants were disappointed when they found out they were randomized to the exercise and medication group. To some extent, this 'anti-medication' sentiment may have played a role by making patients less excited or enthused about their combined exercise and medication program."

He theorized that exercise may be beneficial because patients are actually taking an active role in their own recovery. "Simply taking a pill is very passive," he said. "Patients who exercised may have felt a greater sense of mastery over their condition and gained a greater sense of accomplishment. They may have felt more self-confident and competent because they were able to do it themselves, and attributed their improvement to their ability to exercise. Once patients start feeling better, they tend to exercise more, which makes them feel even better."

Researchers used the anti-depressant Zoloft. This is commonly prescribed anti-depressant known as a selective serotonin reuptake inhibitor (SSRI).

Blumenthal was careful to emphasize that the study did not include patients who were acutely suicidal or had been diagnosed with severe psychotic depression. The subjects who participated in the study were people who desired to find a cure for their depression symptoms and were motivated to faithfully follow the regimens suggested by the research team.

While the Duke University studies are encouraging, the researchers seemed to be left with the impression that the benefits of exercise were largely psychological due to a feeling of self-empowerment and control experienced by the patients. Similar studies conducted at Hull University, the Mayo Clinic, and by other independent researchers theorize that the relief of depression symptoms brought about by regular exercise is possibly the result of actual biological factors in addition to the self-efficacy observed by Duke researchers.

As of the writing of this book, the most prominent theories as to how physical activity dramatically reduces anxiety, stress, and depression symptoms are as follows:

Thermogenic Hypothesis

The thermogenic hypothesis contends that an increase in core body temperature following exercise causes a reduction in symptoms of depression. Increases in temperature of specific brain regions leads to a feeling of relaxation and reduction in muscular tension. This effect seems to be most powerful on anxiety as opposed to outright depression symptoms. This phenomenon may also help explain the beneficial effects of warm baths and saunas on people's emotional state.

Endorphin Hypothesis

This hypothesis focuses on the increased release of endorphins following exercise and their positive effect on depression symptoms. Endorphins are related to a positive mood and enhance an overall sense of well-being.

Monoamine Hypothesis

The monoamine hypothesis currently appears to be the most promising of the proposed biological mechanisms. This hypothesis states that exercise leads to an increase of brain neurotransmitters such as serotonin, dopamine, and norepinephrine. These chemicals are normally lowered in patients suffering with depression. Animal studies indicate that exercise increases serotonin and norepinephrine in vital brain regions. Thus far, human studies have not been conducted due to the difficulty and dangers of performing these clinical tests on people.

The three preceding theories focus on the possible biological explanations for exercise's effects on anxiety and depression symptoms.

The following two theories indicate a psychological cause as noted by the Duke researchers in their studies.

Distraction Hypothesis

The distraction hypothesis suggests that physical activity serves as a distraction from worries and depressing thoughts. The use of distracting activities is a common treatment device in psychological practice today and has been shown to have better results on the management of depression symptoms when compared to more introspective activities like keeping diaries or journals.

Self-Efficacy Hypothesis

Self-efficacy refers to the belief that one possesses the needed skills to complete a task, as well as the confidence that the task can indeed be done with a high expectation of success.

Depressed people often feel helpless to bring about positive changes in their lives and thus have difficulty coping with the symptoms of their depression. This can lead to negative self esteem, prolonged introspections, and a vicious cycle of negative ruminations. These individuals often fall prey to over-analyzing and reliving bad experiences in their minds. This cycle usually ends up producing a warped perception and unrealistic style of thinking. It is now commonly believed that exercise may provide an effective means through which a person can attain a more positive feeling of self mastery.

As can be seen, the effectiveness of regular physical activity on depression symptoms is not in question, even if the reasons for the observed benefits are not fully understood. The important thing for us to keep in mind is that almost all recent research studies have been consistent in their observations and conclusions. Routine rigorous exercise 3–4 times per week is as effective as medications for a large percentage of depression patients.

The Effect of Diet and Supplementation on Depression Symptoms

Regular physical activity and exercise is only one of the natural ways that have been demonstrated to have a positive effect in battling anxiety and depression. Foods high in unhealthy fats as well as large amounts of sugars and caffeine have been shown to increase symptoms of anxiety.

Conversely, foods high in omega-3 fatty acids, vitamin D, amino acids, and antioxidants have been clinically shown to decrease anxiety and depression.

This may help explain why depression is 60 times more common in New Zealand, for example, than Japan. Japanese tend to eat 4–10 times as much fish as many other developed countries around the world. Interestingly enough, studies have shown an almost perfect correlation between the amounts of seafood consumed each year and depression symptoms. Those countries with the highest fish consumption repeatedly demonstrate a lower incidence of depression in their society.

In addition to dietary factors, certain health supplements have been shown to offer relief from the symptoms of anxiety and depression. The most common and documented of these include St. Johns Wort, L-Theanine, omega-3 fish oil capsules (for those not fond of eating fish), SAMe, vitamin D, and Evening Primrose oil, among others.

We will look more closely at these dietary factors and supplement suggestions in future chapters. Both sample diets and guidelines for proper supplementation will be outlined in full detail.

The important fact to keep in mind at this stage is that many people suffering from anxiety and depression MIGHT be among those who can benefit from lifestyle, diet, and supplementation changes. These changes might be able to help them reduce or eliminate a total reliance on medications to deal with their symptoms and enjoy each day with more enthusiasm.

We Know Where We Stand – Now Let's Get Started

In this chapter we have looked at the major physiological and mental changes that are experienced as we pass the human biological peak age of 30 years old. We have looked at how aging affects muscles, metabolism, bones, the heart, blood vessels, lungs, energy, flexibility, mobility, sexual function, and mood. We have cited just a few studies that all show the same results—a well-defined routine of regular exercise, diet, and intelligent supplementation can slow and minimize many factors normally associated with aging.

In the past, "over 40" has often been accepted as the point where we are doomed to begin a rapid decline into being overweight, tired, and plagued with constant aches and pains. Many people passing this midpoint in life feel their best years and achievements are behind them.

For some, this self-fulfilling prophecy has been used as an excuse to justify a choice of lifestyle. For others, they have heard this belief for so long it has simply been accepted as truth.

Today we know this traditional "over 40" mindset is a flawed misconception. Many people in their 40s are reporting being in the best shape of their lives. A number of people in their 50s and 60s (and older) claim to be feeling better than they have in years. Others well past the age of 40 are having some of the biggest business and personal successes of their lives.

Now that we've established that improved fitness is possible at 40, 50, 60, and beyond, it is time to take a closer look at the dietary habits and exercise regimens that will help you realize your goals of self improvement.

Let's get started.

Chapter Three

Your Body Is Much like a Car

Nutrition Class 101

Most people who are overweight eat too much food.

The above sentence may seem like an overly simplistic statement, but most statements of truth really are very simple. If we examine this idea a step further, some people may in fact not be eating an excessive *quantity* of food, but chances are the *quality* of what they are eating is a different story.

Are you skeptical of this bold assertion? A simple example may prove to be an eye opener for some readers. Refer to the photograph below:

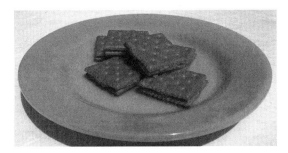

(Photo 3.1) These six crackers contain 210 calories.

The small stack of crackers shown in the preceeding picture contains 210 calories. Certainly this does not appear to be a large quantity of food. However, a 200 lb. man would need to spend 20 minutes walking at 3.3 mph on a treadmill set to a 9 degree incline in order to burn these 210 calories.

Wow—Amazing huh? Hopefully this small demonstration helps reinforce the concept introduced in the opening paragraph of this chapter.

✦ Important Principle ✦

Most people who are overweight eat too much food, or, eat too many low quality foods filled with empty calories.

Food is Everywhere Today and Easily Available to Most

In man's primitive past, survival was largely based on finding and maintaining shelter, water, and food. A large portion of each day was spent hunting and foraging for food. As human society evolved, families often worked on farms where they rose with the roosters at sunrise to work the land and remained in the fields until sunset. During these times, locating and securing sufficient food for survival was often a challenge.

Even as societies developed and people increasingly lived in more populated urban areas where food was purchased from local markets, the cost of food and availability of money often determined how well a person could eat. In fact, during much of the 1700s through early 1900s, excessive weight was viewed not as an unhealthy condition but rather a status symbol representing the wealth of that individual. While excessive weight was rare by today's standards among the working classes, the extremely rich were often rotund and portly.

Today, the availability and cost of food is pretty much taken for granted by the average citizen. Only the very poor in our society still find the quest for food to be a daily matter of life and death. For everybody else, the quest for food is simply a one hour lunch break at work, or a five minute trip to a local fast food drive through on the way home. Even with recent global economic setbacks, food is still relatively cheap compared to yesteryear.

The person living in modern society gives little thought to the idea of hunting or finding food as our ancestors were forced to do. Today food is found on almost every street corner in developed society and even in the small minimarts where we stop to put gasoline in our automobiles. Food for the modern human is no longer what he can grow by his own hand or kill with a spear. Food today is as close as your nearest dollar or ATM/Debit/Credit card.

Eating Today Has Become More about Pleasure and Less about Actual Needs

For most people, the decision on what to eat is guided not by the actual caloric energy needs of their body, but by taste and pleasure. A common scenario seen everyday is the tennis match between a couple or group of people deciding what to eat or where to dine. At this very moment, somewhere in the world at least 30 million people are probably uttering the line, "I don't care. Where do *you* want to eat?" When the decision is finally made, it will most certainly be based on taste, convenience, price, and atmosphere.

This is simply the way food is perceived by the modern human living in a developed society. Over time we have gradually become accustomed to the concept that eating is a social event or habitual custom, as opposed to a necessary act of survival.

"It's twelve o'clock, time for lunch. It's six o'clock, time for dinner." We might not even be hungry, but that is unimportant—it is time to eat! We now live to eat as opposed to eating to live.

Eating Until You are Full is Usually Eating Too Much

Over time, we have gradually acquired an unnatural habit when it comes to consuming food. Many of us eat until we are full. Somehow the idea has developed that we are not supposed to stop eating until we have reached a totally full feeling.

Interestingly enough, this is totally wrong. The feeling of fullness is the body's feedback mechanism to warn us that we have eaten too much. Think of it like the temperature warning light on a car. In the old days, cars used to come with more detailed gauges that showed the precise temperature. Today those informative gauges are often replaced by simplistic "dummy lights." When the warning light comes on, your engine is already too hot. You get no advance notice before reaching that point.

Most scientists tend to agree that it takes about 20 minutes for the brain to receive the message from our bodies that we have reached the point of being full. Combine this with the fact that many people eat on the go or in a hurry, and you can see what happens. People who eat very quickly tend to consume more calories because they take in the food well under the 20 minutes it takes for the brain to get the signal. By the time they receive the message that they are full, they have already eaten more than the amount needed to trigger that original fullness alert.

Several doctors, including Joanne V. Lichten, Ph.D, summarize the scenario as follows: if a person is a rapid eater, it may be beneficial for them to develop a slower pace for dining. Some benefits of eating more slowly include better enjoying the taste of the food and improved digestion.

In her book *Dining Lean: How to Eat Healthy When You Are Not at Home*, Lichten suggests a simple test to see if you are full:
Stand up at some point during your meal and sense how your stomach feels. If you feel comfortable but not overly full when you stand, then you've eaten enough. Doing this simple test can help you avoid the sen-

sation that often occurs at the end of a meal—when you stand up and feel a heavy bloated feeling in your stomach. This is a tell tale sign that you have overindulged.

Interestingly, a number of studies have shown that once people begin eating more slowly, they consume fewer total calories. In some case studies, those simply adopting a practice of eating more slowly lose as much as 20 pounds per year in the absence of any other lifestyle changes.

Author's Note: While the ability to lose some extra pounds as the result of slower eating (and thus fewer consumed calories) is good news, this is only one factor in total fitness. Alone, it is not enough to offset the combination of multiple effects we see from aging. The incorporation of weight training and cardiovascular exercise is still strongly advocated for all the other beneficial reasons discussed in the previous chapter.

Eating 2000 Calories in a Few Large Meals is NOT the Same as Eating 2000 Calories in Many Small Meals

Some people only focus on how many total calories they eat per day. While it is certainly a good idea to be calorie conscience, this is not the whole picture. While we as humans tend to divide our days into 24 hour blocks of time, the human body actually operates in 3–4 hour windows.

Only so many nutrients can be absorbed and utilized in a given segment of time. Any excess food we intake at a given meal must either be eliminated from the body, or retained and stored as body fat. For this reason, eating a single massive meal of 2,000 calories will not be treated the same in your body as five small, light meals of 400 calories scattered throughout the day at 3–4 hour intervals.

In the sections below we will examine how the timing and size of food components are important to consider when planning your daily menu.

The Plague of Modern Western Living

We live in a time where aspects of our society seem to be moving in opposite directions. Our technology evolves each day with advances in computers, science, wireless communication, high density data storage, and the ability to share information and communicate around the globe in mere seconds. You can carry your music collection of 5,000 songs around with you in your pocket. You can talk to friends and family on a smart phone while sharing files and photographs. We live in an era where almost every technology seen on the classic 1960s *Star Trek* TV series has come into your home.

But at this same time, we live in a world that now sees the highest ever rates of obesity, diabetes, high blood pressure, cancer, strokes, heart attacks, sleeping disorders, and mental depression. To be sure, modern medicine has helped improve our ability to survive these maladies, but the frequent use of surgery and medicine seems to have become an over reliance on repairing the car AFTER it has been crashed into a wall, as opposed to avoiding the disaster in the first place.

✦ Important Principle ✦

Prevention Is Better Than Any Known Cure.

At the time of the writing of this book, the Centers for Disease Control and Prevention (CDC) report that 34% of Americans over the age of 20 are overweight.

A few quick facts:

- The rate of obesity (excessive overweight) is now becoming more common in other cultures as western influences in diet and lifestyle become more prevalent and widespread.

- The number of people substantially overweight has been increasing most rapidly in North America, although almost all nations of the world are beginning to also see increases in obesity.

- Obesity is worse in urban settings as compared to rural environments.

- Today, the only part of the world where obesity is not a growing problem is in sub-Saharan Africa.

Other recent studies reveal that over 25% of Americans past age 30 have some degree of insulin resistance which commonly leads to diabetes. Each day we see an increasing number of people contract diabetes. They must usually begin a regimen of measuring blood sugar levels, insulin injections, and diet modifications.

However, research conducted by doctors at Harvard has revealed that 30–60 minutes of regular cardiovascular activity such as walking or using a treadmill combined with a reasonable diet can reduce the chances of contracting diabetes by as much as 40–60%. With this in mind, let's take a look at the basics of nutrition using a unique, entertaining, and original perspective.

The Three Sources of Calories

The title of this chapter states that your body can be thought of as a car. As it turns out, this analogy makes it easy to distinguish the difference between proteins, fats, and carbohydrates and how each of these is important to the body in different ways.

We will now look at the major categories of nutrients and use this information to structure the ideal dietary profile for obtaining and maintaining a healthy lean bodyweight.

Protein

Protein is a nutrient needed by the human body for growth and maintenance. After water, protein is the most abundant molecule in the body. Protein is the major structural component for most of our body, including organs, blood cells, skin, hair, and especially muscle. Proteins also serve as the precursors for enzymes, hormones, immune factors, cellular repair, and other functions essential for life.

In our comparison to an automobile, you can think of protein as being the material from which the fenders, seats, windshield, steering wheel ,and other major components are made. Essentially, the bulk of the car is protein in our analogy.

Proteins contain 4 kcal (calories) per gram. In the absence of carbohydrates, proteins can be utilized by the body for energy, although the mechanism of their digestion for this purpose is not very efficient. Therefore, under normal conditions, the body will choose to use carbohydrates first as a primary energy source. This fact is important to remember as we will see in a few minutes when we discuss carbohydrates in greater detail.

Since protein is needed as a repair and maintenance nutrient, the amount we need to consume daily remains fairly constant based on our lean body weight. By lean body weight, we are referring to what we would weigh if we subtract any excess and undesired fat we may be carrying around our midsection or on our hips and thighs.

Scales are actually almost worthless when it comes to monitoring your healthy weight. The mirror is a much better tool than scales when it comes to determining ideal bodyweight, but for now we need some approximate point to get started.

It is generally accepted that 45–55 grams of protein must be consumed daily to prevent deficiency. Protein deficiency is undesirable since the body will start breaking down muscles and other organs to scavenge the protein needed in cases of severe depletion.

The formula for precisely determining daily protein requirements as per the above guidelines is as follows:

Protein required/day(grams) = Lean Body Weight(kg) x 0.8g/kg

> *Example: For a man with a lean body weight of 90.9kg*
> *Daily Protein need = 90.9kg x 0.8g/kg = 72.7 grams*

For those more comfortable with the American system of pounds, the formula is as follows:

Protein required/day (grams) = Lean Body Weight (lbs) x .364g/lb

> *Example: For a man with a lean body weight of 200lbs*
> *Daily Protein need = 200lbs x 0.364g/lb = 72.8 grams*

The standard guidelines given above were established for the normal sedentary person.

While there is little controversy over these minimum requirements of protein needed to avoid outright deficiency, a debate has raged for years over the ideal amount of protein needed in the daily diet. Two camps continue to argue the advantages and disadvantages of protein consumption at levels greater than these recommended minimum daily requirements.

In the first camp, there are those who feel a higher protein diet can place excess strain on the liver and kidneys. This group also maintains that since proteins are nitrogen-based molecules, excess amounts will break down to ammonia in the body, causing damage to cells as well as loss of vitamin B-6 and calcium.

In the second camp are those who point at a long history of athletes and fitness professionals who routinely follow a diet higher in lean proteins, low in fats, with carbohydrates consumed at just the right levels needed to supply required energy and maintain desired bodyweight. This group points out that in otherwise healthy individuals with no history of liver or kidney ailment, there has been no evidence to date showing any adverse health effects for people consuming as much as 1.5 grams of protein per pound of lean bodyweight.

In fact, many professional strength athletes consume as much as 300 or more grams of protein daily. However, even this second group contends there is no benefit to the normal person consuming levels greater than 1 gram per pound of lean bodyweight, as it is unlikely to be utilized by the body and must be excreted.

At this point, we see we have two recommendations for daily protein intake. Continuing with our 200 lb. individual above, the Recommended Daily Allowance is 73 grams for a sedentary individual, while the sports fitness community feels 200 grams is potentially more appropriate for a person who is somewhat active.

Which recommendation is appropriate for those of us past the age of 40 looking to combine a properly structured diet and exercise routine to slow the hands of time?

Before answering this question, there is one more factor to consider. Research results published in the July 2009 issue of *Clinical Geriatrics* reveal that older people probably need more protein than younger ones.

Why is this? It seems older muscle cells are less responsive to the effects of insulin, a hormone which aids amino acid uptake into muscle tissue. Additionally, the best time for higher protein consumption is in the two hour time window immediately before and after a strength resistance training workout. This timing allows for a positive nitrogen balance so that protein can best be utilized by the muscles for tissue growth.

It is important to stress that resistance training in the absence of sufficient protein will greatly hamper progress and minimize results.

Combining this finding with the recommended protein range above, I recommend a daily diet profile where daily protein intake is 1.0 gram per pound of lean body weight.

Thus, a woman whose desired lean bodyweight is 125 pounds would structure a diet where she consumes 125 grams of protein daily. A man whose desired lean bodyweight is 200 pounds would consume 200 grams of protein daily.

Revising the formula shown earlier to incorporate our revised recommendation for daily protein requirements is as follows:

Protein required/day (grams) = Lean Body Weight (kg) x 2.2g/kg

Example: For a man with a lean body weight of 90.9kg
Daily Protein need = 90.9kg x 2.2 g/kg = 200 grams

For those more comfortable with the American system of pounds, the formula is as follows:

Protein required/day (grams) = Lean Body Weight (lbs) x 1.0g/lb

Example: For a man with a lean body weight of 200lbs
Daily Protein need = 200lbs x 1.0 g/lb = 200 grams

This amount of protein is higher than the minimum recommended value, but well below the level that some fear could be an extra burden on otherwise healthy liver or kidneys. The small surplus ensures sufficient protein is available to overcome the inherent inefficiency of aging muscle cells to transport and utilize protein for muscle growth.

Protein Types
There are different ways to look at protein types. Some people choose to look at protein types in terms of their source (animal versus plant). Others prefer to categorize proteins based upon their amino acid profiles (complete versus incomplete). For our purposes, we are more concerned

with looking at proteins in terms of their biological activity and speed of assimilation.

Our first way of looking at protein is on the basis of bioavailability. Proteins are ranked using a system called the Protein Digestibility Corrected Amino Acid Score (PDCAAS) This ranking is a method of evaluating protein quality based on both the amino acid requirements of humans and our ability to digest and utilize that protein. The PDCAAS rating was adopted by the US Food and Drug Administration (FDA) and the Food and Agricultural Organization of the United Nations/World Health Organization (FAO/WHO) in 1993 as "the preferred 'best'" method to determine protein quality.

The highest rating possible for a protein under this ranking system is 1.00. For the sake of simplicity, one can think of a protein rated at 1.00 as being 100% utilized by the body. By comparison, a food ranked at 0.60 would indicate your body will only utilize 60% of the available protein.

High PDCAAS Protein
Egg whites, whey, soy, and milk (casein) protein all have ranking of 1.00. Beef and soybeans have ranks of 0.92 and 0.91 respectively.

Lower PDCAAS Protein
Most fruits, beans, and other vegetable sources have rankings in the 0.70–0.80 range. Protein found in most cereals, nuts, and wheat grains have a ranking of 0.40–0.50.

Why is the PDCAAS informative and potentially important? If we have determined based on the calculations above that we need to consume 120 grams of protein daily, we could possibly be shortchanging ourselves if our entire diet consisted of only low PDCAAS protein sources. We may consume 120 total grams of protein during the course of the day, but only 50–60 grams may be used by our bodies if they are all low ranked protein types. Designing a diet regimen that includes a fair share of higher quality proteins is the goal with the program described in this book.

Our second way of looking at protein types is based upon the speed in which they are digested and used by the body. Proteins from whey, milk, eggs, vegetable, and meat sources are all digested and assimilated by the body at different speeds. Professional athletes will go to great lengths to select different protein sources at various times of day to try to maximize strength or recovery from hard training.

For our purposes, we do not need to go into such detail in thinking about which proteins we wish to eat during the day. We will simplify our view of protein speeds into two types.

Fast Proteins
Whey proteins are a perfect example of fast proteins. These are best consumed immediately before and after your exercise routine since they quickly supply amino acids to your muscles to begin the recovery process after a good weight resistance workout. These whey proteins are easily and conveniently available in the forms of protein shakes and flavored drinks.

Recent studies also suggest that whey protein may be of additional benefit to seniors since it is more easily digested and absorbed, thus overcoming some of the limitations and inefficiencies of our aging digestion systems. Individuals allergic to milk or related dairy products may need to avoid whey products.

Slow Proteins
These proteins should make up most of your other meals during the rest of the day. These include milk, eggs, meats, and the various vegetable proteins. These are not absorbed into the bodily as rapidly as whey protein, but they provide a supply of amino acids and a feeling of fullness for several hours.

I should stress that our classification of protein types is both informative and useful, so that we can design a diet plan that is optimized to give you the best results possible. But in the final analysis, your top concern is to consume the appropriate amount of protein each day as calculated for your desired bodyweight. Our discussion of protein quality and speed is for the purpose of giving you an extra edge, optimizing your diet plan, and getting the most benefit from each calorie you consume.

Protein Sources
Having now determined both the appropriate amount and types of protein that should be consumed daily, what are suggested food sources to obtain that protein? As you may have guessed, like most things in life, not all proteins are created equal.

Some proteins are considered complete proteins as they contain nine of the essential amino acids needed by the body *(Histadine, Isoleucine, Leucine, Lysine, Methionine, Phenylalanine, Threonine, Tryptophan, and Valine)*. These amino acids are called "essential" since the body is unable to synthesize them itself and thus they must be consumed from external food sources.

Other protein sources are considered incomplete as they are missing some of these key amino acids. As a general rule, it is easier to find complete proteins from animal sources. But select vegetable sources also provide a full amino acid profile.

Animal sources for complete proteins include:
• Meat
• Poultry
• Seafood/Shellfish/Fish
• Eggs
• Cheese
• Milk

When you consume these foods, you take in all the essential amino acids in a single food source.

Plant sources for complete proteins include:
- Buckwheat
- Soybeans
- Quinoa
- Hempseed

Most people who eat a variety of both plant and animal based foods typically do not have to worry about whether they are consuming complete proteins. The natural variety in their daily diet will typically take care of their needs.

Pure vegetarians who never consume animal-based foods of any kind and may not daily consume the full proteins indicated in the plant source list above usually need to be more conscientious of what they eat in order to prevent a protein shortage. A common practice for pure vegetarians is to consume a wide variety of vegetable sources during the course of the day. By eating such a wide variety of different plant-based sources, one food normally contains what another may be missing. By the end of a day, this protein combination usually overlaps enough to ensure that all the essential amino acids have been acquired.

Let's take a quick look at a variety of common foods along with their protein and major nutrient content:

Food	Calories	Protein	Carbs	Fat
Meats and Fish				
Beef (95% lean), 4 oz	282	44	0	10
Beef Round (eye), 8 oz	448	77	0	13
Canadian Bacon, 51 grams	60	11	1	1.5
Cheese (cheddar), 1 cup	455	28	1	37
Chicken Breast, 8 oz	248	52	0	4
Eggs, 1 Jumbo	90	8	0	6
Filet Mignon, 8 oz	494	62	0	25
Ham (deli), 7 oz	290	42	2	12
Milk (whole), 1 cup	146	8	13	8

Food	Calories	Protein	Carbs	Fat
Pork (lean), 7 oz	223	42	0	5
Shrimp, 6 oz	170	36	0	2
Turkey Breast, 8 oz	304	54	0	6
Venison Steak, 7 oz	310	64	0	4
Vegetables and Plants				
Asparagus, 10 spears	32	4	6	0
Broccoli, 1 cup chopped	33	3	6	0
Buckwheat, 1 oz	96	4	20	1
Carrots, 1 cup chopped	52	1	12	1
Celery, 1 cup chopped	18	1	3	0
Corn, 1 cup	127	5	27	2
Green beans, 1 cup	131	2	7	0
Hempseed, 30 grams	174	11	2	14
Potato (baking)	165	5	37	0
Quinoa, 185 grams	222	8	39	4
Soybeans, 1 cup	254	22	20	12

Note – Protein, Carbohydrates, and Fat are expressed in grams

As can be seen from this sampling of popular foods, it becomes apparent why it is much easier to get desired levels of protein from meat and fish sources as compared to strictly vegetables. However, it should be noted that complete plant source proteins like hempseed, quinoa, and soybeans pack quite a bit of protein-punch for those leaning towards a vegetarian diet.

Protein Utilization

From the last two sections relating to protein, you should now have an idea how much protein you require each day, and also an idea of some protein-rich foods that personally appeal to you.

There is one more thing to consider. We must look at the best way to consume that protein each day.

Research reveals that the human body is only able to digest and absorb 30–45 grams of protein per 3–5 hour time window. Obviously there is some variability in this figure, as we would expect a 200 lb individual lifting heavy weights to be able to utilize more protein in this time frame compared to a 125 lb individual sitting in an office meeting. However, this figure of 30–45 grams is a well accepted range that is very useful for us to know.

Why is this important information? Let us again use our 200 lb individual as an example. We have determined that this person should aim to consume 180–200 grams of protein daily under the diet guidelines being explained in this book. If the human body is only able to utilize 30–45 grams of protein at one time, this means at least 5 meals must be consumed during the course of the day to ensure the needed amount of protein can be digested and utilized by the body for repair and maintenance. For this person, the goal would be to consume 30–40 grams of protein at each of 5–6 meals during the day in order to promote assimilation while also reaching the daily desired target of 200 grams. As you may expect, a smaller individual may only require 4–5 small meals to reach their daily protein goals given this same limitation of only being able to utilize 30–40 grams of protein at one time.

If a person were to only eat one big meal for the day and then starve for the next 23 hours, they would face a lose/lose situation. They would fail to absorb the recommended amount of protein for the purpose of tissue growth. At the same time, they would probably be adding to their adipose fat reserves and placing excess demand on their body's excretion systems. This is a bad situation all the way around and should be avoided.

This is probably not the first time you have heard it said that eating 4–6 small meals per day is better for weight control and your health than consuming 2 or 3 larger meals. Our examination of protein utilization may help explain from where this recommendation was derived. It is not just some theoretical fad or trendy idea that sounds good, rather it is based on physiological fact. It is simply the way the body works.

✦ Important Principle ✦

The human body can only utilize 30–45 grams of protein inside a 3–5 hour window of time.

For this reason, it is advisable for most people to eat 4–6 small meals spaced out over the course of the day as opposed to only a few large meals.

As we move ahead and examine fats and carbohydrates in the diet, we will see this concept of multiple small meals get reinforced again with even more emphasis.

Most important to keep in mind regarding our discussion of protein is:

- We want to consume an amount of protein (in grams) each day that is approximately equal to our desired lean bodyweight in pounds.

- For example, an individual aiming to weigh 135 pounds should be consuming about 135 grams of protein daily.

- Since the body can only utilize 30–45 grams of protein at a time, it is necessary to divide the daily menu into 4–6 small meals as opposed to the 1–3 large meals that have become common in our modern day urbanized Western civilization.

Now, we will take a look at the next major source of calories.

Fats

Fats play a vital role in maintaining healthy skin and hair, insulating body organs against shock, protecting nerves, maintaining body temperature, and promoting healthy cell function. Some vitamins such as A, D, E, and K are fat-soluble and can only be digested, absorbed, and transported via fats. Dietary fat is also the source for essential fatty acids which are needed for normal glandular activity. The adrenal and sex hormones require the presence of fatty acids in order to maintain proper levels.

Fat also serves as a buffer against some diseases and toxins. When a hazardous substance reaches unsafe levels in the bloodstream, the body can often partially dilute or equilibrate the offending substance by storing it in fat tissue. This action helps to protect vital organs from immediate critical damage until the dangerous substance can be metabolized and/ or removed from the body by mechanisms such as excretion, urination, bloodletting, and hair growth.

In our comparison to an automobile, you can think of fat as being similar to the motor oil in your engine. The oil is essential to lubricate the engine and allow it to run, but we do not require a massive amount of it in our diet.

Fats contain 9 kcal (calories) per gram. In the 90s, dietary fats were labeled as the greatest evil in the world. They were almost shunned like a social disease or leprosy. Many new fat-free diets and foods became the fad of the day, with all kinds of chemical substitutes introduced to take the place of fats. Despite the popularity of these fat-free diets, the general population continued to grow in girth and the numbers of Americans categorized as obese continued to climb. Why?

In order to maintain an acceptable taste in their products, many manufacturers simply added more sugars to replace the fats that had been removed. Twenty years later, we see the results. More people than ever before in our society are battling not only excess weight, but also diabetes. The lesson learned from this era of dietary experimentation is that fats are not pure evil. Most fats can be healthy and in many cases are essential.

The one exception is trans-fats. Trans-fats do indeed seem to be a product spawned by the Devil himself and dumped on mankind as a form of dietary plague. We will discuss this more later.

While fats supply over twice the caloric energy of protein or carbohydrates, they must undergo a longer digestive process before they are ready to provide energy following a carbohydrate metabolism pathway. As we will see in the next section, carbohydrates do a much more efficient job of providing the body with readily usable fuel. In terms of energy, fats are really most valuable as a form of stored energy reserve, but strictly speaking, they are not a necessity in the diet as far as a fuel source is concerned.

Fats are more extensively stored within the body than carbohydrates and may be converted into fuel when the body's carbohydrate reserves are depleted. This metabolic phenomenon is exactly what occurs when a person goes on a diet, fasts, or is exposed to extremely cold weather. When the stored carbohydrate reserves in the liver are exhausted, the body's fat reserves are metabolized for a new supply. When fats are called upon to be converted to energy, they split into fatty acids and glycerol. Glycerol is then converted to either glucose or glycogen. At this point, the usual carbohydrate metabolism pathway takes over to produce needed energy from the glucose and glycogen.

It is important to clarify that fat reserves in the body do not simply come from the fat that is eaten in the diet. When excess carbohydrates are eaten, they are converted by the body into fat and stored. In this way, the body can store and use fat without having a large amount of fat in the diet. These fat deposits can be thought of as a "carbohydrate reserve bank." When carbohydrates are available, they are used first. When there are no carbohydrates available, withdrawals are made from the fat reserves as necessary. This process of forcing the body to utilize fat reserves as a source of energy is the underlying objective of any weight loss diet plan.

Although fat within the body can serve as an important energy and heat source, strictly speaking, it is not an essential or even preferred source for bodily fuel.

✦ Important Principle ✦

Do not confuse Dietary Fat with Body Fat.

Dietary Fats are an essential component of the daily diet that are needed for healthy skin, hair, and other organs as well as assisting with absorption and utilization of certain vitamins. Body Fat is the accumulation of adipose tissue on the body resulting from an excess consumption of calories from all sources (fats, proteins, and carbohydrates).

Since fat is primarily needed only for a specific number of bodily functions and secondly as a back-up energy reserve for carbohydrates, the amount we need to consume daily remains fairly constant based on our lean body weight. This is a similar situation to what we saw earlier with protein.

Also, since we are humans living in a modern world, and are not animals that hibernate for months at a time, we normally do not require (or desire) accumulating excess body fat to aid in surviving the winter or long bouts of starvation. It is generally accepted that a minimum of 20–30 grams of fat need to be consumed daily to prevent deficiency and allow for proper utilization of fat soluble vitamins. As a rule, the medical and scientific community contends that the maximum amount of total dietary fats that should be consumed daily regardless of body weight or physical size is around 100 grams. In actual practice, most people will fall in the range of 40–65 maximum grams per day. This amount will equate to approximately 15–35% of their daily calorie consumption coming from dietary fats.

This wide range results from differing opinion on the amount of dietary fats needed in the daily diet and the variability that results from using total calories as the starting point for calculating macronutrient needs. To be more precise and individualistic, we need to determine the amount of fat required for a given lean body mass and not over simplify the calculation by only considering fat intake as a percentage of calories consumed.

Why is this? If a person overestimates their total daily calorie consumption, they will likewise run the possibility of over-calculating and consuming too many fat grams using the conventional "% of calories" logic.

As was the case when we calculated protein requirements above, it is my opinion that using the common practice of determining macronutrient requirements (protein, fats, carbohydrates) as a percentage of total calories is a somewhat backwards approach. Instead of trying to guess or estimate the total number of calories needed per day and then back calculate the amount of protein, fat, and carbohydrates that should theoretically be consumed—why not structure our dietary profile based on the specific body we want to build?

If for example, we desire to have a lean, strong, and healthy body of 150 pounds bodyweight, and dietary science tells us the appropriate amount of protein and fats needed to nourish that size body, then why not design our diet with that specific goal in mind as opposed to limiting ourselves to estimates and rules of thumb?

With this thought in mind, our formula for determining daily fat requirements is as follows:

Fat/day (grams) = Lean Body Weight (kg) x 0.44g/kg

Example: For a man with a lean body weight of 90.9kg
Daily Fats needed = 90.9kg x 0.44g/kg = 40.0 grams

Again, for those more comfortable with the American system of pounds, the formula is as follows:

Fat/day (grams) = Lean Body Weight (lbs) x 0.20/lb

Example: For a man with a lean body weight of 200lbs
Daily Fats needed = 200lbs x 0.20g/lb = 40.0 grams

As this example calculation shows, we get a suggested fat intake amount of 40 grams for our 200 pound test subject. This calculated result falls within the accepted range of 30–100 fat grams to be consumed daily, but is specifically calculated for this specific body size/weight. We did not simply back calculate from an estimated total calorie consumption (that may be wrong to begin with).

The reason this approach of calculating dietary needs appears to be more precise and accurate for our purposes will become even more apparent when we discuss carbohydrates in the next section. But for now, let's continue learning about fats.

Fat Types
There are generally considered to be four main types of dietary fat, although some dieticians prefer to subdivide these groups into deeper detail. For our purposes, the four major groupings are sufficient to understand what we should eat and what we should avoid when designing our personal dietary menu. Although we may refer to a food as a source of saturated fat or a source of trans-fat, it is never really that simple in real life.

In nature, most fat sources are a combination of more than one fat type. One type often far exceeds the others in proportion such that we can safely categorize it based on the predominant fat source. For example, olive oil is often referred to as a source of monounsaturated fat, but also contains small concentrations of polyunsaturated and saturated fats. With this in mind, the four major groups of fats are:

Monounsaturated fat

This type of fat is commonly found in a variety of natural foods and oils. Studies show that eating foods rich in these fats improves blood cholesterol levels, possibly decreasing your risk of heart disease. Research also shows that these fats may support insulin levels and control blood sugar readings, which can be helpful for those wrestling with type 2 diabetes.

Polyunsaturated fat

This type of fat is found mostly in plant-based foods and oils. Evidence shows that eating foods rich in polyunsaturated fats can improve blood cholesterol levels, which can decrease the risk of heart disease. Some studies indicate that these fats may also help decrease the risk of type 2 diabetes.

One type of polyunsaturated fat, omega-3 fatty acids, have become popular in recent years. Research indicates these omega-3s may be especially beneficial to your heart and appear to decrease the risk of coronary artery disease. Some studies indicate they may also protect against irregular heartbeat and can lower blood pressure readings.

Saturated fat

This type of fat comes primarily from animal food sources, although there are a number of non-animal sources such as palm oil that are also high in saturated fats. Studies since the 1950s have shown that heavy consumption of saturated fats raise blood cholesterol levels and low-density lipoprotein (LDL) cholesterol levels. Elevated cholesterol and LDL levels can increase the risk of cardiovascular disease. Saturated fat may also increase the risk of type 2 diabetes.

Trans-fats

This type of fat does occur naturally in some animal source foods, but in the modern diet, most trans-fats come from commercial food processing via the hydrogenation of unsaturated fats. Hydrogenation is the chemical process used to make oils solid by forcing hydrogen atoms into the polyunsaturated fatty acid molecules found in most vegetable oils.

Partially hydrogenating the oil makes it semi-solid, but creates the dreaded trans-fats. Fully hydrogenating the oil turns the liquid oil into a harder solid, much like a saturated fat. Fully hydrogenated fats are not often used in cooking since they are hard and solid at room temperature. Partially hydrogenated fats on the other hand, are semi-solid at room temperature. Some brands of margarine and shortening are made with partially hydrogenated oils.

✦ Important Principle ✦

Trans-fats are also referred to as "partially hydrogenated oils." Avoid these like the plague.

"Fully hydrogenated oil" does NOT contain trans-fat, but is very dense and saturated. While these fats may be healthier by comparison to trans-fats, they are still less healthy than the various unsaturated and natural liquid fats.

The process of partial hydrogenation creates fats that are easier to cook with and less likely to spoil than naturally occurring oils. Research studies show that more than any other type of fat, synthetic trans-fat can increase unhealthy LDL cholesterol and lower healthy high-density lipoprotein (HDL) cholesterol. This can increase the risk of cardiovascular disease.

In mankind's simpler past, animal-based fats were really the only trans-fats people regularly consumed. But today that situation has dramatically changed. The largest amount of trans-fat consumed today comes from various chemically hydrogenated vegetable oils. These partially hydrogenated fats have displaced natural solid fats and liquid oils in most common large scale food production applications. You will find hydrogenated oils used extensively in both the fast food and snack food industries (including most fried foods, and store shelf baked goods).

You may be wondering why these fats which are known to be so detrimental to our health are also so prevalent today. The answer is simple. They are cheap and they have a very long shelf life. Partial hydrogenation increases product shelf life as much as ten times compared to natural oil, while also decreasing refrigeration requirements. Many baked foods require semi-solid fats to suspend solids at room temperature. Partially hydrogenated oils are perfect for this use as they have the right consistency to replace animal fats like butter and lard at lower costs without the risk of spoilage.

There continue to be numerous theories as to why trans-fats are so harmful to human health. A prevailing theory contends that the addition of extra hydrogen to the molecule prevents the body from being able to properly break down the fat in the body. In effect, the chemically modified fat is not something our body's biochemistry was ever designed to digest. Perhaps this is not so surprising—we can't digest motor oil either.

So how do you identify trans-fats when examining products on your store shelf? If a package simply lists "hydrogenated oil," without expressly stating whether it is partially or fully hydrogenated, it may not be trans-fat free. Sometimes the terms "hydrogenated" and "partially hydrogenated" are used interchangeably. If the package clearly states that it contains "fully hydrogenated oil," then it will be trans-fat free.

In recent years, stricter labeling laws have made it easier to quickly identify the presence of trans-fats in foods since they usually now have their own separate listing under the Fats section.

Fat Sources
From our description of fat categories, you may have already guessed that our goal is to eat mostly monounsaturated and polyunsaturated

fats in our diet. We can also consume a small amount of saturated fats, but even this is not desirable whenever it can be avoided. Saturated fats should be kept below 15 total grams per day maximum.

Tran-fats (partially hydrogenated oils) are in a class all their own. These should simply be avoided. There is nothing beneficial about them and they bring nothing but harm.

Let's take a quick look at a variety of sources for dietary fats:

Foods containing primarily Monounsaturated fat (good)
Olive oil
Canola oil
Sesame oil
Avocado
Nuts (almonds, cashews, pistachios, peanuts, and natural peanut butter)

Foods containing primarily Polyunsaturated fat (good)
Corn oil
Cottonseed oil
Safflower oils
Sunflower seeds and Sunflower oil
Flaxseed and flaxseed oil
Soybeans and Soybean oil
Seafood
Omega-3 fats *(Fatty, cold-water fish, such as salmon, sardines, and tuna are rich in preformed omega-3s. Enteric coated capsules are also available for those who dislike the taste of fish but still wish to benefit from this excellent and healthy dietary fat).*

Foods containing primarily Saturated fat (not so good)
Fatty meats
Full fat cheeses
Full fat ice cream
Whole milk
Coconut oil
Palm oil
Palm kernel oil

Foods containing Trans-fat (partially hydrogenated oils) (BAD)
Microwave popcorns
Stick margarine
Shortening (though many brands are now changing formulations)
Many fast food items
Many brands of store bought cookies, crackers, and snacks that have long shelf lives.

Fat Utilization

When structuring our daily eating routine, we should treat fats pretty much the same way as proteins. This means it is advisable to divide your fat consumption throughout the course of the day, eating a portion of fat with each meal. In practice, this equates to about 10–15 grams of fat consumed at each meal or every other meal. This spacing out of fat consumption improves the efficiency of digestion and helps to prevent accumulating excess fat calories where we don't want them.

What does 10–15 grams of fat look like? Due to the wide range of fat sources available, the best way to answer that question is to read the labels of the foods you are actually eating. But here are some basic examples and guidelines that should give you an idea:

Food	Calories	Total Fat	Sat-Fat	Trans-fat
Almonds, 1 oz	160	13	1	0
Macadamia nuts, 1.2 oz	260	27	4	0
Peanuts, 1 oz	160	14	2	0
Walnuts, 1 oz	200	20	2	0
Olive Oil, 1 Tbsp	120	14	2	0
Peanut Oil, 1Tbsp	120	14	2.5	0
Sesame Oil, 1 Tbsp	130	14	2	0
Microwave Popcorn (bag)	510	36	7.5	13.5
Snack Crackers (6 pack)	210	12	2.5	0
Ramen Noodles (3 oz)	380	14	7	0
Fast Food "Super Burger"	790	39	17	2
Large Fast Food Fries	500	25	3.5	0

Note- Fat values expressed in grams.

Only basic fat information shown.
Other calories result from proteins and carbohydrates.
An ounce of nuts fits roughly in the palm of your hand.
No specific brand names or menu items are specified. Pseudonyms have been used.

In the list above, you may have noticed the high fat and calorie content found in the microwave popcorn and fast food combo meal consisting of a "super burger" and large fries. The combined fat content found in just these three items alone is almost enough to fulfill our dietary fat requirement for 2–3 days. Yikes!

At first glance a person may not think a burger and fries at lunch and a bag of popcorn in the evening while watching TV seems like an excess amount of food. But when we take a closer look at the nutritional profile of items such as these, it quickly becomes apparent why so many people in our society today have a problem with excess weight gain and cardiovascular health.

In daily practice, you will find cooking lean protein meals using a small amount of the healthy fats will provide an appropriate amount of dietary fat at that meal. At other times during the day while you are on the go, a handful of nuts like almonds, cashews, or peanuts will provide 15 grams of fat in between your major prepared meals.

It is almost unheard of that anyone in our modern society suffers from a dietary fat deficiency. While you may find yourself needing to give thought to the best ways to get more lean protein in your diet, fats will pretty much take care of themselves. If anything, with fats we need to be sure we don't get more than enough. In a society that seems to rely heavily on fats and salt for flavoring, it is very easy to get too much fat and sodium without realizing it.

At the end of this chapter, we will look at some sample daily meal plans to help put this dietary information into useful perspective.

Now let's take a look at the last of the three macronutrients.

Carbohydrates

In the previous sections dealing with protein and fats, we made reference to carbohydrates. You may be wondering why we saved this nutrient and calorie source for last. We saved carbohydrates for last because this is the area where you will have the most variability in your dietary planning.

In our comparison to an automobile, you can think of carbohydrates as the gasoline you put in the tank so your engine can run and your car can move. We already established the fact that protein and fat intake should be relative to your body size and weight and thus will not vary greatly from day to day. On the other hand, carbohydrate intake will vary to a much greater extent depending upon your activity levels. Carbohydrate consumption will also be the calorie source that gets decreased or increased depending upon your weight loss (or gain) goals.

Carbohydrates contain 4 kcal (calories) per gram. The primary function of carbohydrates is to provide energy for the body, brain, and nervous system. The enzyme amylase helps break down carbohydrates into glucose (blood sugar), which is used as the primary fuel in the body.

Most organs in the body can use protein or fat for energy if carbohydrates are not available. However, the brain requires some small amount of carbohydrate (available as glucose-blood sugar) to function properly. You may have heard of ultra-low carbohydrate diets where less than 20 carbohydrates are consumed daily while protein intake is increased. This diet is effective at shedding weight quickly by placing the body in a state of ketosis. Ketosis is essentially a controlled form of starvation where carbohydrate intake is cut so drastically that the body has no choice but to deplete glycogen reserves in the liver and begin burning fat for fuel. By simultaneously consuming an increased amount of protein, muscle scavenging is prevented and the body more readily burns away fat reserves. Many times people on such diets complain of feeling a bit "mentally fuzzy." No doubt, the dulling of the mental senses these people experience is probably due to the decreased level of carbohydrates readily available for the brain to use as fuel.

As a rule, the medical and scientific community maintains that the average person should get 40–60% of their daily calories consumption from carbohydrates. As with our calculations for protein and fats above, I feel we should be more precise, scientific, and individualistic in our calculations. It is fine to know that roughly 40–60% of your daily calories should come from carbohydrates. But that assumes you know the right number of total calories you should be eating in the first place.

Are you trying to lose weight? Are you trying to gain weight? Are you a sedentary person watching TV 10 hours per day? Are you an active person playing tennis and riding a bike 20 miles per week?

As we explained earlier, if a person overestimates their total daily calorie consumption, they will likewise run the possibility of over-calculating and consuming too many carbohydrates using the conventional "% of calories" logic. Again, it is my opinion that using the common practice of determining protein, fat, and carbohydrate requirements as a percentage of total calories is a backwards approach. We have already demonstrated a very precise manner of calculating target amounts of protein and fats.

Our method is fine-tuned specifically for any desired body size and weight. We will now calculate an appropriate level of carbohydrates that will serve as a base level for our future dietary adjustments. With this thought in mind, our formula for determining baseline carbohydrate requirements is as follows:

Carbs/day (grams) = Lean Body Weight (kg) x 3.3g/kg

Example: For a man with a lean body weight of 90.9kg
Daily Carbs needed = 90.9kg x 3.3g/kg = 300 grams

Again, for those more comfortable with the American system of pounds, the formula is as follows:

> **Carbs/day (grams) = Lean Body Weight (lbs) x 1.5/lb**
>
> *Example: For a man with a lean body weight of 200lbs*
> *Daily Carbs needed = 200lbs x 1.5g/lb = 300 grams*

As this example calculation shows, we get a suggested daily carbohydrate amount of 300 grams for our 200 pound test subject.

This calculated value has a slightly different meaning than the calculation we did earlier to determine suggested protein and fat intake. While the values we calculated for protein and fat are intended to be a relatively solid target level with minimal variation, the value we receive when calculating carbohydrates can be quite variable.

As mentioned earlier, it is the changes you make with your carbohydrate consumption that will be used to lose, maintain, or gain weight. Carbohydrates are the nutrient you will be increasing or decreasing in order to adjust your daily calorie consumption.

This adaptive dieting will be used to help you reach and maintain your personal goals. Think of this calculated value for daily carbohydrate consumption as a baseline starting point from which you may have to make changes to suit your personal metabolism, activity levels, and weight control goals.

Carbohydrate Types
In Chapter One, I promised not to make this book an all encompassing text on everything known to man regarding diet, nutrition, and exercise. But a certain degree of technical information is important when it comes to some topics. Understanding and mastering these basic concepts will make it much easier to incorporate the information in this

book into your daily routine. Knowledge is power, and having that knowledge will make food profiling become second nature to you.

Since carbohydrates are the part of the diet where most of your daily variation will occur, they are also the nutrient that requires a deeper understanding. Not all carbohydrates are the same. This is an important fact to remember.

Different forms of carbohydrates cause different reactions in the body. Some are able to enter the bloodstream rapidly and provide a quick energy boost, while others supply a slow and steady level of energy. The type, amount, and rate of digestion/assimilation of different carbohydrate sources determine the level of blood glucose in your system and the amount of insulin released by the pancreas.

Insulin is the all important hormone responsible for enabling excess blood glucose to be stored in muscle cells and in the liver (as glycogen). When the glycogen levels in the liver are full, any excess blood glucose not needed for immediate energy is converted to fat and stored in the body.

Those aware of the growing problem of diabetes today are probably already familiar with the relationship between blood sugar and insulin. Diabetes is basically a metabolic disease in which a person has high blood glucose (blood sugar) because insulin production is either inadequate, or the body's cells do not respond properly to the insulin which is present.

For those fortunate enough not to be touched by diabetes, or those a bit rusty on human endocrinology, here is a brief explanation of the basic carbohydrate-insulin-blood sugar-glycogen process: all forms of carbohydrates are digested in the intestine to form glucose. This produced sugar is then transported around the body via the blood and taken into cells to be converted into energy. Insulin is secreted by the pancreas to control the rate of cell glucose uptake. Excess glucose is converted into glycogen, which as we mentioned above is stored in the liver or in fat around the body. If the body requires more energy, another hormone, glucagon, is secreted by the pancreas to convert the stored glycogen back into glucose. This glucose is then released back into the bloodstream so that with the help of insulin, the cells can take up the glucose to release the energy they need.

The glucose or sugar metabolism of the body is a continuous cycle of glucose, insulin, and glucagon reactions. The slower the release of glucose and hormones, the more stable and sustainable the energy levels of the body. It is generally accepted that the more processed the carbohydrate, the faster the glucose will enter the blood. This results in less stable energy levels in the body.

We are all familiar with kids who experience a "sugar buzz" after eating a bowl of sweetened cereal. You may also know diabetics who make a habit of carrying hard candy with them in the event they misjudged their insulin injection for the day and go into diabetic shock. When a person experiences diabetic shock, they are suffering from an excessively high insulin level. Ingesting a quick-acting sugar like that found in hard sweet candy can quickly help restore the proper sugar balance in their system.

With this basic explanation in mind, carbohydrates are typically divided into two major classes:

Simple Carbohydrates
This category of carbohydrates is made up of monosaccharides and disaccharides. These two words are simply fancy ways of saying either the simplest form of sugar or a molecule that is a combination of two of these simple sugars.

A monosaccharide can't be hydrolyzed or broken down any further to form a simpler sugar. Examples include glucose (dextrose) and fructose (commonly called fruit sugar). These simple forms of sugar tend to taste very sweet. While dextrose is quickly absorbed into the intestine and rapidly spikes blood sugar and insulin levels, fruit sugar is digested quite a bit more slowly and has less of a dramatic effect on blood sugar.

A disaccharide is made up of two simpler sugars (monosaccharides). They also taste sweet and tend to have a relatively fast absorption rate in the body. Examples of these types of carbohydrates include lactose (*glucose + galactose*), maltose (*glucose + glucose*), and sucrose (*glucose + fructose*). Each of these three sugars impacts your blood sugar and insulin levels in different ways, with maltose being absorbed the fastest and lactose the slowest.

Complex Carbohydrates

Complex carbohydrates are sometimes also referred to as polysaccharides. These complex carbohydrates are formed by the bonding of several chains of mono and disaccharides. More commonly people will think of these as being starches, glycogen, and cellulose.

Although there are a few exceptions, you can think of complex carbohydrates as those that digest slower and provide sustained energy. These types of carbohydrates also have less dramatic impact on blood sugar and insulin levels. Complex carbohydrates in the form of dietary fiber are not readily digested by the human body, but provide many benefits in addition to physically aiding the digestion process.

Dietary Fiber has been shown to :

• Normalize bowel movements.
Fiber increases the weight and size of your stool and softens it. A bulky stool is easier to pass, decreasing the chance of constipation. For some, fiber may provide relief from irritable bowel syndrome.

• Help maintain bowel integrity and health.
A higher fiber diet may lower your risk of developing hemorrhoids, and small recesses or pouches in your colon (diverticular disease).

• Lower blood cholesterol level.

Soluble fiber found in beans, oats, flaxseed and oat bran may help lower total cholesterol levels by lowering low-density lipoprotein, or "bad" cholesterol levels in the blood. Some studies have shown that sufficient fiber in the diet can reduce blood pressure and inflammation which is good for heart health.

• Help control blood sugar levels.

Soluble fiber can slow the absorption of sugar. For people coping with diabetes, this can help improve blood sugar levels. A diet that includes insoluble fiber has been associated with a reduced risk of developing type 2 diabetes.

• Aid in weight loss.

High-fiber foods generally require more chewing time, which gives your body time to register when you are no longer hungry. This is helpful for those who tend to overeat due to fast eating. A high-fiber diet also tends to make a meal feel larger and last longer, so you stay full for a greater amount of time. Higher fiber diets also tend to be less "calorie dense," which means they contain fewer total calories for the same volume of food.

As you may have already guessed, complex carbohydrates should comprise the majority of your daily carbohydrate consumption. While this rule of thumb is a good one to follow, there is one more aspect of carbohydrates we need to examine to have a full picture.

Glycemic Index

From the information above, you may be under the impression that all one needs to do is eat complex carbohydrates and avoid simple sugars and everything will be fine. This is actually a good rule to follow, and loosely speaking this advice will serve you well 80% of the time. But it is not 100% accurate. Why is this?

As with most things in life, there are exceptions to almost any rule and using the logic that all simple sugars are fast digesting, and all complex carbs are slowly absorbed is oversimplifying things slightly. Some simple carbohydrates like fructose (fruit sugar) have a relatively minor impact on blood levels, while a complex carbohydrate like maltodextrin actually raises blood sugar and insulin levels rapidly.

So what is a person to do? In the early 1980s, doctors at the University of Toronto conducted research to determine the best foods for diabetics. From these studies, they developed a system called the Glycemic Index. The Glycemic Index is the measurement of glucose (blood sugar) level increase from different carbohydrate consumption. Foods raise glucose to different levels. The GI estimates how much each gram of available carbohydrate (total carbohydrate minus fiber) in a food raises a person's blood glucose level following consumption as compared to the identical consumption of pure glucose. By definition, glucose is given a glycemic index of 100. Other foods are rated relative to glucose in terms of their impact on blood sugar levels.

This is a much more exacting and scientific way of looking at the impact of different foods as opposed to simply lumping them into the two categories of simple versus complex carbohydrates. This system was originally developed to aid diabetics in food selection, but it has proven to be an accurate and refined method of selecting carbohydrates for all people.

For diabetics, the proper selection of carbohydrate sources can potentially mean life or death. For everyone else, the proper selection of carbohydrates can help prevent unwanted weight gain and even the potential development of diabetes.

Simply summarized, the higher a food's Glycemic Index number the more dramatic an impact it will have on blood sugar and insulin levels. In daily practice, our goal is to eat mostly carbohydrate sources with a

Glycemic Index of 69 or lower, while limiting the consumption of food with a GI above 70.

The list below shows the Glycemic Index for a selection of popular foods:

Food Source	Glycemic Index
Dextrose	111
Glucose	100
Maltodextrin	100
Popular Hi-Carb Sports Drink	100
Baked Potato (no skin)	98
White Rice	89
Instant Oatmeal	83
Rice Cake	82
Jelly Bean Candy	80
White Sandwich Bread	75
Watermelon	75
Bagel (plain white bread)	73
Baked Potato (with skin)	69
Whole Wheat Bread	68
Raisins	66
Pineapple	66
Cantaloupe	65
Instant Oatmeal (high fiber type)	55
Corn	54
Oatmeal (steel cut variety)	52
Brown Rice	50
Banana	47
Apple	38
Yam	35
Low fat milk	30
Black beans	30

The Glycemic Index numbers shown in most reference lists are for that food in a solitary state. When combined with other food components, the effective glycemic index may be altered higher or lower. For example, consuming carbohydrates in the presence of proteins will often slow their rate of absorption. The relative rate of absorption will not change however between different foods. This means that a sugar sweetened soda consumed with a lean protein will still have a higher glycemic index than a bowl of high fiber oatmeal eaten with a lean protein.

Carbohydrate Sources

As far back as the 1970s (if not earlier), many experts in the fitness and nutrition world were voicing concerns over the rampant spread and increasing amounts of refined sugar in the Western diet. I recall reading a book written in 1977 by legendary bodybuilder Franco Columbu. In it, he strongly proclaimed *"sugar is my idea of slow poison. If we poured sugar down the gas tanks of our cars the way we pour it down our systems, we would shut down Detroit."*

The reason this quote has stuck in my mind is because of the analogy we have been making that your body is much like a car. Ironically, the city of Detroit referenced by Mr. Columbu in this quote is not in great shape today either.

In the last section we explained the Glycemic Index. When choosing carbohydrate sources, we want to structure the majority of our diet around lower glycemic foods. These types of foods will not spike blood sugar levels nor excessively elevate insulin into our system.

✦ Important Principle ✦

Eat mostly low glycemic and complex carbohydrates while keeping simple refined sugars to a minimum.

Low glycemic foods provide long term energy and maintain stable blood sugar and insulin levels in your system.

By contrast, heavy consumption of high glycemic foods and simple sugars wreak havoc on the body in many ways. Energy levels climb and crash as a result of rapid glucose absorption when eating mostly simple sugars. Over time the constant spiking and crashing of sugar and insulin levels can promote excess weight gain and the onset of diabetes. Simple sugars are also more prone to lead to tooth decay, vitamin loss, and nervous conditions.

When structuring our daily diets, we want to include foods like oatmeal, brown rice, whole wheat breads and pastas, vegetables, whole fruits, and black beans. We want to limit our consumption of "empty calories" like doughnuts, sugar-coated cereals, jellies, jams, potato chips, crackers, cookies, ice creams, salad dressings, sodas, deep fried starchy foods, and products made with white flour, high fructose corn syrup, and large amounts of white sugar.

With today's FDA food labeling requirements, it is easier than ever to evaluate a food at a glance to see if it is appropriate to meet your desired needs. But to get familiar with some popular foods, here is a small list of items with their total carbohydrate, fiber, and sugar content:

Food	Calories	Total Carbs	Fiber	Sugar
Good Choices:				
Broccoli, 1-stalk	98	20	9	4
Brown Rice, 1/2 cup	150	33	4	0
Green Beans, 1 cup	27	6	3	1
Oatmeal (instant hi-fiber), 45gr	160	29	6	1
Rice Cake (caramel), 1 cake	50	11	0	3
Sweet Potato, 1 large	162	37	6	12

Food	Calories	Total Carbs	Fiber	Sugar
Limit Consumption of these:				
Cereal (popular sweetened), 3/4 cup	110	23	1	15
Corn chips snack, 28 grams	140	19	2	0
Crackers (cheesy), 30 grams	150	19	0	0
Potato Chips, popular brand, 28 gr.	160	15	0	0
Ramen Noodles, 42 gr.	190	26	2	0

Note: Carbohydrate values expressed in grams.
Only basic carbohydrate information shown.
Other calories result from proteins and fats.

The first question a person may ask when looking at the list above is why certain foods like corn chips, cheese crackers, and potato chips are on the limited consumption list. Their profile looks pretty good based on the information shown. While we are focusing on carbohydrates in this section, one must always remember that the various food nutrients do not exist alone in a vacuum.

Using the potato chips as an example, the full nutritional profile including fats and protein reads as follows:

Potato Chips	(Serving Size = 1 oz/28 grams.) (Approx 17 chips)
Total Fat	10 grams
Saturated Fat	3 grams
Sodium	200 mg
Total Carbohydrate	15 grams
Dietary Fiber	0 grams
Sugar	0 grams
Protein	2 grams

We see that 90 of the calories in these potato chips come from fat. That equates to 56% of the calories in a potato chip coming from fats. Skinless potatoes as we know from the list above have a high glycemic index of 98, however, in the presence of large amounts of fats, the starch from potatoes is more slowly absorbed which lowers the effective glycemic index.

The result here is that only 17 potato chips provide 25% of the total fats we have calculated are required by the majority of average-sized individuals in a single day. The carbohydrates from potato chips have an effective glycemic index of around 55–60. So enjoy your occasional small snack of potato chips. Life is too short to deprive oneself of all pleasures or to live like a Spartan. Just don't make a regular meal out of potato chips and large sugary sodas.

Carbohydrate Utilization

We stressed earlier that your body works much like an automobile. The utilization and spacing of carbohydrate consumption further demonstrates this point. If you are planning a trip from Florida to California, you can't simply fill up your tank one time with 97 gallons of gasoline and drive non-stop for the full 2,800 miles. You must stop along the way to refuel as you burn the gasoline.

Your body works in much the same way. Biologically, the digestive system works in 3–4 hour windows. This means when you are thinking about what you want to eat now, you should also be thinking about what you plan to be doing in the next three to four hours.

If you try to cram all 97 gallons of gas into your car at one time to make the entire trip to California, the excess gas is going to spill out on the ground. Likewise, if you consume 2500 calories in a single meal to try to last for the next 24 hours, your body is going to do two things:

1. Try to eliminate what it can't use. This of course places more burden on your digestive and elimination system. Think of the classic feeling associated with the post-holiday feast.
2. The excess calories will spill out, but not on the ground. They will spill out on your hips, thighs, and around the middle.

Earlier we stressed that protein and fat intake should be evenly spaced throughout the day. Carbohydrate intake should be based on the level of activity you have planned for the next three to four hours following that meal. In daily practice this means most people will eat more carbohydrates in the morning upon awaking and gradually decrease the amount of carbohydrates they consume with each meal during the day. The last meal of the night, consumed just hours before bedtime, should usually be the lowest carbohydrate meal of the day.

An example of such a meal may be fire-grilled shrimp and steamed broccoli. In this example, we have a high protein source that will aid in muscle and tissue recovery while we sleep, but the carbohydrates from broccoli are almost exclusively fiber.

Having just read these last few paragraphs, the first thought that may cross your mind is how the habits of our Western society seem to run 180 degrees opposite to this advice. In our society, the idea of three meals per day has been the norm for decades. Often this means a quick, small breakfast grabbed on the go. Lunch may be a fair to medium-sized meal. For the majority of people, the evening dinner meal is the biggest feast of the day.

Yes, this is tradition. Yes, this is ingrained habit. Yes, most of us were raised with this mindset. But No, it is not the way the human body works.

✦ Important Principle ✦

Ideally, our goal is to regulate daily carbohydrate consumption based on our planned activity level for the next 3–4 hours.

In practice, this means your highest level of carbohydrate consumption would be immediately before and after exercise at the gym. Conversely, for most people who are less active in the evening as they prepare for bed, the amount of carbohydrates consumed should dramatically decrease as they relax in front of the TV or prepare for bed.

This practice of planning carbohydrate consumption to synchronize with levels of activity is especially important for those fighting to lose or maintain weight. Any excess calories remaining at the end of each 3–4 hour window of time following a meal are more readily converted to body fat in those individuals cursed with a metabolism that makes weight gain frustratingly simple.

Those blessed with a fast metabolism who never gain weight no matter how much they eat can be a bit more flexible in these eating schedules as far as weight control is concerned. However, the idea of eating 4–6 small meals per day as opposed to 2–3 large meals is still advised for everybody. Smaller meals mean less stress is placed on the digestion and elimination systems to handle the volume of food consumed.

Weight control is certainly a challenge for those of us 40 and over, but it is not the only concern we must keep in mind. We must also help our stomachs, intestines, bile ducts, pancreas, liver, colon, and other organs as much as we can. All of these body parts have been with us since we were born and experience a decrease in operational efficiency with the passage of time.

Water

The human body contains approximately 67% water. Depending on body size, the actual percentage can vary from 55% to 78%.

To function properly, the body needs to remain hydrated. Preventing dehydration requires the consumption of 1–7 liters of water per day. This wide range in daily water requirement results from the variability of body size, activity level, temperature, humidity, perspiration, diet, and other factors.

When a person fails to intake enough water (either from food or liquid drinks), several symptoms will begin to occur. The body's early response to dehydration is thirst. It is important to note that when you get thirsty, your body is already in a mild state of dehydration and is trying to trigger you to increase water intake.

Another early sign of dehydration is decreased urine output as the body acts to try to conserve further water loss. At this stage, the urine will become concentrated and a darker yellow in color.

As the level of water loss increases, more symptoms can become apparent. The following is a list of the most common signs and symptoms of dehydration:

- Dry mouth
- Decreased urine output
- Reduced tear production
- Sweating may stop
- Muscle cramps
- Nausea and vomiting
- Heart palpitations
- Lightheadedness
- Weakness

In the case of severe dehydration, confusion and weakness will occur as the brain and other body organs receive less blood. Eventually if the body is not hydrated, coma, organ failure, and death will result.

Conversely, it is possible to drink too much water and create a form of water intoxication. In this condition the excess water overwhelms the body's kidneys and offsets osmotic balance in the cells. In normal daily practice, it is extremely difficult for a person to place themselves into a state of hyponatremia (water intoxication). We normally see people suffer this condition only when they enter some foolish contest or otherwise intentionally try to consume a large volume of water in a short period of time. In other words, it is almost impossible to over-hydrate by accident. A person must really make an effort to overwhelm his system with excess water.

How much water should we drink daily? We have all heard the common rule of thumb to "drink eight 8-ounce glasses of water daily". This is not a bad guideline to follow as a rough rule of thumb. But it is only that—a rough rule of thumb. By that I mean that if you have gone all day long working in the hot sun, and only had a single 6-oz glass of liquid, chances are you might be entering a state of dehydration. By the same token, if it is late in the day, and you have had 8–9 glasses of water over the past 16 hours, and your urine is clear or pale yellow in color, chances are you are in good shape.

As was the case with our calculations for protein, fats, and carbohydrates it is nice to have a rough guideline to get us in the ballpark, but we should really listen to our own bodies and customize consumption to our specific needs.

I support the idea of being sure you drink at least eight 8-ounce glasses of liquid daily as a starting point. However, I add three conditions that will help you fine tune this approximation to be sure you are staying hydrated:

- Your urine should be a pale yellow color. A dark yellow color is normally a sign that the urine is becoming too concentrated with waste materials due to dehydration.

- When in a hydrated state, you should find that you need to urinate every few hours.

- You should start your day by drinking a full glass of water upon waking in the morning. After eight hours of sleep, you have lost water through cellular activity and expiration. Re-hydrating first thing in the morning is a perfect way to get your system kick-started and your mouth, throat, and esophagus lubricated and ready for the first meal of the day.

Personally speaking, I have noticed that not drinking enough water adds to a feeling of lethargy and loss of energy. Water itself does not contain any calories or energy producing compounds, but it is the "universal solvent" that all the cells in our body use to carry out their chemical reactions and elimination processes. Being a living creature that is approximately 70% water, it makes logical sense why a lack of water hampers our function.

Tap Water, Bottled Water, or other source?

85% of Americans get their drinking water from public water supplies. In order to prevent illness or other biological contamination, public water supplies are normally chlorinated. The use of chlorination is important since many organisms found in raw water supplies can be immediately hazardous to human health. However the germ-killing benefits of chlorination are not without their own negative side effects.

Chlorine can react with naturally occurring organic compounds found in the water supply to produce compounds known as disinfection byproducts. The most common of these are trihalomethanes(THMs) and haloacetic acids (HAAs). Since most of these compounds have been shown to be potentially carcinogenic, strict drinking water regulations have been introduced across the developed world. These regulations require regular monitoring of the concentration of these compounds in the distribution systems of municipal water systems. The World Health Organization has stated that they feel the risks to health from these byproducts are extremely small in comparison with the immediate risks associated with inadequate disinfection.

There are also other concerns regarding chlorine, such as disagreeable taste and odor. Additionally, at various times during the year, most municipalities must "shock" their distribution systems with excess chlorination to cleanse the system and overcome any resistance that may have formed in biological organisms. During these times, the levels of disinfection byproducts are greatly increased.

In the last few decades, the bottled water industry has grown to an estimated $60–70 billion industry. This growth is amazing when one considers that the cost of bottled water per gallon is higher than the controversial cost of gasoline in the United States. The reasons people are willing to pay for bottled water are numerous, but include natural disaster preparation, desire to reduce chlorine and fluoride consumption, convenience, and a perception of better purity. Of all these reasons, it is probably the idea of better quality that motivates most people to pay for bottled water.

Is this idea of better quality accurate? Sometimes Yes. Sometimes No.

Many people are surprised to learn that, as of the writing of this book, the regulations governing bottled water are less stringent than those that govern public tap water in most parts of the world. In recent years, there have been numerous reports of bottled water being sold that is in fact only tap water, water from untested springs, and even river water collected downstream from industrial sites. Statistically speaking, most bottled water suppliers are reputable. But one must keep in mind that you can never be 100% certain of the true source of the water you are drinking when you open a plastic container of bottled water.

When buying bottled water, I often advise people to choose Purified or Distilled water over those that advertise "Spring Water" or some other "Natural Source." Why?

If the water is identified as purified or distilled, you know it was treated in some way prior to being bottled regardless of the source. Often when a bottled water vendor advertises spring water or some other natural source, they are assuming the water was pure and pristine and no form of purification was needed. This may be an accurate assumption—but maybe it is not.

Home Distillation
Taking all the information above into consideration, I have personally distilled water in our own home for years. During the 1990s, I was a cofounder and vice president for one of Florida's largest environmental

testing laboratories. During that time I worked with the EPA and Florida Department of Health and Florida Department of Environmental Protection on various regulations and methodologies.

As a chemist working in the industry since 1985 and the technical director of our environmental laboratory for nine years, I reviewed well over 100,000 laboratory testing reports. I have had an opportunity to see firsthand the chemical compositions of raw water supplies, public finished drinking water supplies, and bottled waters from all across the United States. This firsthand knowledge prompted me to make the decision to begin distilling water in our own home.

As mentioned earlier the World Health Organization (and most other health organizations like the EPA and FDA) contends that the potential effects from chlorination byproducts are far less risky to human health than the immediate illness or death that would occur from drinking untreated water. I agree with that statement.

Certain biological organisms can kill you in days. Cancer may or may not ever develop in an individual. Public water supplies do need to be disinfected for obvious reasons. To date, alternatives to chlorination have not been as successful or widespread—so most people not on private wells and relying on public water supplies will need to deal with chlorination.

Just how much potential health risk do these disinfection byproducts of chlorination introduce? The debate rages. For every study that shows no definitive health hazards from the long term consumption of low level THMs and HAAs, there are other studies that indicate an increased incidence of cancer.

My feeling is, why take a risk when it is so easy to avoid this issue altogether? With home distillation, you can have the best of both worlds. If you are on a public water supply, you can feel secure in knowing the chlorination process is killing any pathogens or germs that would cause immediate intestinal distress, illness, or death. But by home distilling your own water, you can remove the disinfection byproducts before you drink. This way you get all the benefit and none of the potential harm.

Many companies now manufacture small self-contained distillation units for the home that are easy to use. Different models exist that are able to produce different volumes of water based on a family's size and needs. Even the smallest of these units are usually able to produce 5–6 gallons per day.

People sometimes have two concerns about distilled water:

1. "Is drinking distilled water healthy? Somebody told me with all the minerals removed the water would strip my body of nutrients."

Water is not your main source of minerals like sodium, magnesium, potassium, etc. Once foods and water are combined in your stomach, your body does not know where the minerals came from. Imagine you just ate a few potato chips and drank a glass of water. In your stomach the chewed potato chips are being churned and mixed with the water you drank. The sodium from the potato chips is now dissolved in the water. Your body does not care (or have any way of knowing) if that sodium was originally supplied by the water or from the potato chips.

2. "I did not think distillation removes all impurities?"

There is some validity to this concern. As a rule, distillation does a better job removing materials that do not evaporate such as sediments, heavy metals, salts, etc. Being a volatile organic compound, some disinfection byproducts can carry over in the steam during the distillation process, but two factors make this more of a concern in theory than actual practice.

First, most of these THMs and HAAs do not retain an affinity for water and will boil away in the heating process and vaporize. Secondly, distillation units normally include a carbon filter near the end of the process to trap any traces of organic compounds that may have survived the distillation process. In either event, you can rest assured you have removed an estimated 95% of these types of contaminants.

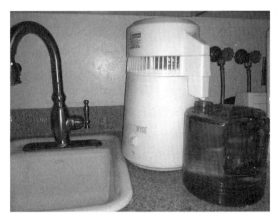

(Photo 3.2) A home water distillation unit such as this model made by Waterwise is able to produce 5–6 gallons of purified water daily.

Considering that our body is roughly 70% water and we need to consume 60–70 ounces of water per day to remain hydrated, I feel the water we drink should be as pure as possible. Distilling your own water at home gives you some peace of mind knowing exactly what you are drinking. Are you always on the go? You can fill containers and be your own personal bottled water factory.

Vitamins & Minerals

One could write a full length book about the discovery, history, and importance of vitamins and minerals. In fact, many such books have been written on this very topic. Very detailed descriptions of vitamins and minerals are also easily found on the internet. There are tons of great links that describe recommended daily allowances as well as possible problems that may result from both deficiency and overdose of each.

For our needs and purposes, there is no need to delve too deeply into this area. For us, it highly advisable to take a quality multivitamin and mineral supplement daily. The better supplement companies today offer formulations specifically designed to meet the needs of men and women over the age of 50.

Putting It All Together

Okay, we have finished looking at Protein, Fats, Carbohydrates, Fiber, Water, Vitamins, and Minerals. That is really the entire scope of dietary intake for the human animal. All the various foods and drinks we take in each day are just assorted combinations of these primary building blocks.

Theory and scientific knowledge are good, but how do we put all this information to practical use? We will do that now.

Below we will create a sample daily meal plan for two individuals using the information explained above.

One plan will be for a person with a desired bodyweight of 125 pounds. The second plan will be for a 200 pound individual. From these examples, you will get an idea how to create your own daily eating regimen.

First, we must calculate how much of each macronutrient we need for each of these individuals. Of course, this is not something that needs to be done everyday. Once you know the amounts of protein, fats, and carbohydrates you should be eating for your desired body size, those values remain fairly constant. The creativity is introduced when you think about the exact meals you plan to eat each day.

125 Pound Individual

Using the formulas described earlier, we can determine the desired levels of Protein, Fats, and Carbohydrates to be consumed daily:

Protein =   Weight x 1.0 = **125 grams**   (33.9% of total calories)

Fats =   Weight x 0.2 = **25 grams**   (15.25% of total calories)

Carbs =   Weight x 1.5 = **188 grams**   (50.85% of total calories)

Total Calories = 1475

We also know we want to divide our protein and fat intake fairly evenly over 4–6 meals during the day while consuming the majority of carbohydrates before and after periods of most intense physical activity. We will plan for 4–6 meals for the day.

This means we will be aiming to get approximately 25 grams of protein and 5 grams of fat at each meal. Our carbohydrates will be approximately 38 grams at each meal, with those values being shifted higher around the time we exercise or engage in other physical activity. Likewise, they will be lower when we only plan to watch TV, sit behind a desk at work, or are preparing for bed.

200 Pound Individual

Using the formulas described earlier, we can determine the desired levels of Protein, Fats, and Carbohydrates to be consumed daily:

Protein =   Weight x 1.0 = **200 grams**   (33.9% of total calories)

Fats =   Weight x 0.2 = **40 grams**   (15.25% of total calories)

Carbs =   Weight x 1.5 = **300 grams**   (50.85% of total calories)

Total Calories = 2360

As with the previous individual, we know we want to divide our protein and fat intake fairly evenly over 4–6 meals during the day while consuming the majority of carbohydrates before and after periods of most intense physical activity. We will again plan for 4–6 meals during the course of the day.

This means we will be aiming to get approximately 40 grams of protein and 8 grams of fat at each meal. Our carbohydrates will be approximately 50–60 grams at each meal, with those values being shifted higher around the time we exercise or engage in some other activity. Likewise, they will be lower when we only plan to be watching TV, sitting behind a desk, or preparing for bed.

Sample Meals

Following are sample meal plans for the 125 lb and 200 lb individuals we just calculated values for above. These should serve to demonstrate a practical application of the ideas and principles discussed in this chapter.

The different meals of the day alternate between shaded and non-shaded rows in the tables below. Note each sample plan features 5–6 meals during the day. Each meal is spaced approximately 3–4 hours apart. Except where specifically identified otherwise, beverages are water, unsweetened tea, lemon water, or diet sodas in these examples. We aim to eat our higher amounts of carbohydrates and protein before and after exercise.

As was already mentioned before, this kind of detailed mathematical breakdown is not something you need to do everyday. However, if this is your first time seriously evaluating food nutrients because you realize you need to make changes to your dietary habits, this could be a useful exercise for a week or two.

✦ Helpful Hint ✦

Alternating low carbohydrate protein shakes with regular food makes it easy to obtain desired protein intake while keeping overall calories lower.

For those designing a daily eating plan consisting of 5 small meals, this would translate to 3 meals of regular food separated by 2 protein shakes between morning and night.

The average person structures their eating habits around the same 20–30 foods and the same 12–20 recipes. Certainly there is some variety outside of this habit when we go to a new restaurant or visit a foreign

125 Pound Individual – *Meal Plan 1*			
PROTEIN-gr	CARB-gr	FAT-gr	MEAL DESCRIPTION
11	1	2	1 Slice Canadian Bacon
6	13	12	1/2 English Muffin & Cheese
2	26	0	Orange Juice
1	11	0	Rice Cake
30	45	4	Grilled Shrimp & Rice
2	22	0	1 Peach X-large
34	30	2	Protein Shake
30	23	8	Ginger Chicken & Broccoli
Protein-gr	Carb-gr	Fat-gr	Total Calories
116	171	28	1400
Protein-cal	Carb-cal	Fat-cal	
464	684	252	
% of Cal.	% of Cal.	% of Cal.	
33.14%	48.86%	18.00%	100.00%

125 Pound Individual – *Meal Plan 2*			
PROTEIN-gr	CARB-gr	FAT-gr	MEAL DESCRIPTION
6	1	5	Hard Boiled Egg
4	24	9	Wheat Toast & Butter
2	26	0	Orange Juice
34	30	2	Protein Shake
2	14	10	Tossed Salad w/dressing
30	45	1	Grilled Chicken & Rice
34	30	2	Protein Shake
Protein-gr	Carb-gr	Fat-gr	Total Calories
112	170	29	1389
Protein-cal	Carb-cal	Fat-cal	
448	680	261	
% of Cal.	% of Cal.	% of Cal.	
32.25%	48.96%	18.79%	100.00%

200 Pound Individual – *Meal Plan 1*

PROTEIN-gr	CARB-gr	FAT-gr	MEAL DESCRIPTION
7	32	3	Oatmeal-maple flavored
18	27	5	2 Eggs & OJ
9	16	16	Rice Cake & Peanut Butter
34	30	2	Protein Shake
4	38	1	2 Apples
30	45	4	Grilled Shrimp & Rice
8	45	2	Oat Bar
34	30	2	Protein Shake
30	23	8	Ginger Chicken & Broccoli
34	8	2	Lo-Carb Protein Drink

Protein-gr	Carb-gr	Fat-gr	
208	294	45	
Protein-cal	Carb-cal	Fat-cal	Total Calories
832	1176	405	2413
% of Cal.	% of Cal.	% of Cal.	
34.48%	48.74%	16.78%	100.00%

200 Pound Individual – *Meal Plan 2*

PROTEIN-gr	CARB-gr	FAT-gr	MEAL DESCRIPTION
10	41	5	Mueslix Cereal & Milk
2	26	0	Orange Juice
2	11	0	Rice Cake-Caramel Flavor
34	30	2	Protein Shake
8	39	4	Quinoa Bar
35	31	7	Salad-Jerk Chicken-Cheese
34	30	2	Protein Shake
3	31	8	2 Windmill Cookies
44	33	18	4 oz Steak & Potato w/Butter
34	8	2	Lo-Carb Protein Drink

Protein-gr	Carb-gr	Fat-gr	
206	280	48	
Protein-cal	Carb-cal	Fat-cal	Total Calories
824	1120	432	2376
% of Cal.	% of Cal.	% of Cal.	
34.68%	47.14%	18.18%	100.00%

country. But in everyday life, most people fall into a routine of revolving their eating around the same foods.

Until you get a solid grasp of the nutritional content of common foods, you may desire to apply this calculation on your own meals in order to discover what you are really consuming. Some people find themselves surprised (or shocked) when they learn just how much they have really been eating in the past.

I assure you—in no time at all, you will be able to evaluate food automatically without going through this exercise. You will soon be able to instantly evaluate your dietary needs for the next 3–4 hours and select your upcoming meal "on the fly."

Losing Weight Diet Modifications

Being aware of the trend towards increased obesity we see in most of the developed world today, it is probably safe to say 75% of the people reading this book will be interested in losing excess body fat (losing weight).

Losing weight and being in good health both rely on the same three factors: Genetics, Diet, and Exercise. We can't do anything about our inherited genetics, but we do have control over the other two factors.

Diet more than anything determines weight control. Why do I say this? If you recall, earlier in the book we showed a picture of just a few crackers that added up to a total of 210 calories. We also explained how it would take a large man 20–30 minutes of fast walking on an inclined treadmill to burn those same 210 calories.

A pound of fat equals roughly 3,500 calories. This means 3,500 calories is a "magical" number when it comes to losing a pound of body fat. If you think of your body like a checking account, you need to withdraw 3,500 calories from your body's fat bank before you will lose a pound of undesired bodyweight.

There are only two ways to create this deficit of calories that will allow your body to shed excess pounds. You must either expend more energy to burn those 3,500 calories or reduce calorie consumption enough to deplete surplus glycogen and force your body to pull from its fat reserves for energy. 3,500 calories might seem like a lot, but if you spread it out over a week, it amounts to a reduction of only 500 calories per day.

Let's compare the option of slightly reducing calorie consumption each day to that of trying to "burn off" excess calories while continuing our same food consumption. The list below shows the calories typically burned for a variety of physical activities:

Activity	Calories Expended Per Hour
Climbing	400-900
Cycling	250-700
Dancing	200-400
Golf	300
Hi-Intensity Cardio	600-1100
Running	800-1000 (depending on speed)
Sawing Wood Logs	420
Skating	300-700
Skiing	600-700
Soccer	550
Swimming	300-700 (depending on stroke)
Walking (slowly)	115
Walking (briskly)	565
Walking (treadmill)	700-800 (with incline and brisk pace)
Weight Training	600

Knowing we need to create a deficit of 3,500 calories in order to burn and lose a single pound of body fat, the question is raised: "Is it easier to eat 500 less calories per day for a week, or saw wood logs for over eight hours to lose one pound of fat?"

Often in life, there is no single solution for any problem. We often find a combination of factors work to help us achieve a desired goal. This synergy is also at work when it comes to our health and weight control goals. To be certain, weight resistance training and cardiovascular exercise burn calories and help with weight loss, but a smart diet is the more effective factor. The combination of both physical activity and diet is that much better.

To a large degree, my advocacy for weight resistance training is more focused on helping maintain strength, flexibility, and mobility. There is, of course, the weight control benefit of burning calories and enhancing our Basal Metabolic Rate as we discussed before. But as we see from the chart above, it takes six hours of weight training to equal the fat loss realized from a 500 calorie reduction in our daily diet.

Our cardiovascular exercise is intended to keep our heart, lungs, and blood vessels as healthy as possible. Yes, there is also the added benefit of extra calorie expenditure, but again, it would take over thirty hours of walking around the block to equal the weight loss of simply cutting 500 calories out of your diet each day.

The bottom line lesson here is that most foods are densely packed with energy. It is easier to avoid consuming excess calories than it is to try to burn them off later.

✦ Important Principle ✦

It is much easier to avoid eating excess calories than it is to try to burn them off later.

So how do we best cut those 500 (or more) calories per day? We have learned that once we have established the amount of Protein and Fats we need for a desired lean bodyweight, those values should remain fairly consistent in our daily diets. Carbohydrates are the flexible variable we modify up or down as needed to adapt to differing energy requirements and to modify our weight.

Below I have made a few small changes to Meal Plan 1 that we originally constructed for a 200 lb individual. You will note there has been very little change in the total protein and fats consumed, but the carbohydrate intake has been reduced by 146 grams.

This is approximately half of our normal carbohydrate consumption. Total calories have been reduced by 584. This dietary reduction, combined with our regular level of physical activity, will translate into 1–2 pounds of fat loss per week.

In fact, this meal plan is one I personally used when I reduced my own bodyweight from 236 to 210 over a period of 16 weeks at age 43. This translated to 1.6 pounds lost per week.

This is also consistent with the healthy weight loss of 1–2 pounds per week we expect with a carefully structured exercise and diet regimen. My actual fat loss was probably greater than a simple reduction of 26 pounds since muscle size was also being built and increased at the same time. It may be possible that actual fat loss was a much as 30 pounds, but 4 pounds of muscle mass was added during this same time, resulting in the measured net weight change of 26 pounds.

I still use this kind of diet anytime I notice my midsection getting a little puffy and the mirror reveals the return of love handles.

It is often easy to slightly modify your favorite dishes to lower the overall carbohydrates. Try eating grilled chicken or shrimp over lettuce or steamed/chopped cauliflower instead of rice. Drink unsweetened ice tea or lemon water instead of sugar-loaded sodas. We have used a diet modification example here that is designed to lose 1–2 pounds per week when combined with exercise.

PROTEIN-gr	CARB-gr	FAT-gr	MEAL DESCRIPTION
Modified Meal Plan 1 (for Weight Loss) for 200 lb Individual			
7	32	3	Oatmeal- maple flavored
18	5	5	3 Eggs & Lemon Water
9	16	16	Rice Cake & Peanut Butter
34	8	2	Lo-Carb Protein Drink
2	19	0.5	1 apple
30	45	4	Grilled Shrimp & Rice
34	8	2	Lo-Carb Protein Drink
30	23	8	Ginger Chicken & Broccoli
34	8	2	Lo-Carb Protein Drink

Protein-gr	Carb-gr	Fat-gr	
198	164	42.5	
Protein-cal	Carb-cal	Fat-cal	Total Calories
792	656	382.5	1830.5
% of Cal.	% of Cal.	% of Cal.	
43.27%	35.84%	20.90%	100.00%

Serious Weight Loss Strategy

The principles discussed above are rock solid and honest. However, each of us is different. We may have inherited favorable or unfavorable genetic traits. We may have certain allergies or other dietary restrictions that we must follow to deal with a health condition. Whatever the case, your results will guide you in making the modifications needed when it comes to controlling your weight.

Are you not losing at least one pound per week? Then you need to evaluate your diet.

Are you getting the right amount of protein and fats per day relative to your desired body size, but still not losing weight? Chances are you need to further reduce your carbohydrate and sugar consumption if the weight is not disappearing.

Have you been reducing caloric intake as directed above, but still not losing weight? Perhaps your physical activity is not properly stimulating muscle fibers to keep your Basal Metabolic Rate up to par.

Those needing to lose a substantial amount of weight or coping with challenging genetics may find they need to reduce total carbohydrates to as low as 30–50 grams per day. These carbohydrates must be in the form of complex, low Glycemic Index foods.

For example, a 43 year old associate of mine was approximately 50 pounds overweight. In order for him to lose this undesired body fat, he followed a diet and exercise routine as described in this book for six months. In his particular case, he relied mainly on fibrous carbohydrates like broccoli, green beans, celery, lima beans, and spicy grilled chicken or ultra-lean beef for the mainstay of his diet. He only ate a small serving of rice or potatoes once every two weeks on a designated "cheat day."

If you have a large amount of weight to lose and/or have historically found it very difficult to lose weight regardless of the diet plan followed, then you most likely need a very low carbohydrate meal plan to obtain the results you want.

As we discussed earlier, the only way to lose body fat is to deplete excess carbohydrate reserves and force the body to begin metabolizing fat to generate the energy it needs. If a person with a slow metabolism continues to consume carbohydrates even at a simple "maintenance" level, the body is never going to be forced to start breaking down fat reserves and making withdrawals from its "carbohydrate bank."

At the risk of being repetitive, I will again stress the concept that your daily requirements for protein and fat do not vary regardless of your weight loss (or gain) goals. Your daily protein and fats consumption is based on the desired lean bodyweight you wish to be. Once you have calculated the ideal amounts of protein and fats required to nourish that desired body size, you do not alter those daily amounts. *Only carbohy-*

drates are dramatically modified to meet your goals for losing or gaining weight.

As we have done before, I will provide some examples of this "Ultra-Low Carb" concept in real use. Below is a sample eating plan for a large man trying to reduce his size and weight downwards to a lean and tight 200 pounds. You will notice the amount of protein and fats being consumed daily have not been altered from our other meal plans.

*Ultra-Low Carb Weight Loss Meal Plan for 200 lb Individual*			
PROTEIN-gr	CARB-gr	FAT-gr	MEAL DESCRIPTION
25	2	22	4 Large Eggs
24	3	1	Lo Carb Protein Shake
50	10	0	Chicken Breast & Green Beans
24	3	1	Lo Carb Protein Shake
24	3	6	4 oz Lean Beef & Lettuce
24	3	1	Lo Carb Protein Shake
47	11	1	9oz Shrimp & Broccoli
Protein-gr	Carb-gr	Fat-gr	TOTAL
218	35	32	CALORIES
Protein-cal	Carb-cal	Fat-cal	CONSUMED
872	140	288	1300
% of Cal.	% of Cal.	% of Cal.	
67.08%	10.77%	22.15%	100.00%

Many times people think losing weight requires near starvation, but a look at this meal plan shows how the proper selection of foods can be sufficiently filling, flavorful, yet still low in carbohydrates and total calories.

Now let's take a closer look at the "secret" of low carbohydrate dieting by introducing another useful concept.

The 5 Net Carbohydrate Rule

For individuals trying to lose significant weight with a low carbohydrate diet plan, it is suggested to keep Net Carbs under 5 grams at each meal. Following this simple rule will optimize your weight loss results.

A Net Carbohydrate is defined as the total carbohydrates excluding fiber content.

The formula is as follows:

Net Carbohydrates (grams) = Total Carbohydrates – Fiber

Example: 1 cup of Chopped Broccoli contains:
6 total carbohydrates and 2 grams of fiber.
Net Carbohydrates (grams) = 6 – 2 = 4 grams

Since fiber tends to have a minimal effect on blood sugar levels, and is not normally digested and absorbed, it is not a carbohydrate source that contributes to excess weight gain. On the contrary, fiber is actually important in maintaining a normal and healthy elimination process.

Here is an example of how a nutrition label may look when you are shopping for low net carbohydrate foods:

Nutrition Facts

Serving Size 1 slice 43 grams   Servings Per Container   20
Amount Per Serving
Calories 35   Calories from Fat 25

		% Daily Value
Total Fat	2.5 g	4%
Saturated Fat	0g	0%
Trans Fat	0 g	
Cholesterol	0 mg	0%
Sodium	100 mg	4%
Total Carbohydrate	9g	3%
Dietary Fiber	9g	40%
Soluble Fiber	< 1 g	
Sugars	< 1g	
Protein	3 g	

Looking at this product label, you can see all 9 carbohydrates are fiber. Therefore this would be considered a "Net Carb Zero" food.

This example actually comes from a low carbohydrate bread which is made using oat fiber, egg whites, and other healthy ingredients. This would be an excellent choice for a person preparing a low carbohydrate meal that calls for a single slice of bread.

When designing an Ultra-Low Carb meal plan for weight loss, you should still follow the same routine of eating 5–6 meals per day. These meals should still be spaced at 3 hour intervals.

Eating no more than 5 net carbs (10 total carbs) at each meal will add up to a total of only 30–60 total carbohydrates per day. This total daily carbohydrate amount matches the definition of low carb dieting outlined at the beginning of this section.

In the next example, we will look at an Ultra-Low Carb meal plan for a person aiming for a lean and fit body weight of 150 pounds. For this example, I have incorporated the 5 Net Carbohydrate Rule concept. I have included the Net Carbs for each meal in parenthesis beside the total carbohydrate number.

In this example, you will notice the amount of Protein and Fats consumed each day has not changed from what a non-dieting 150 pound individual would eat. Only the carbohydrates have been reduced to aid in weight loss. In order to optimize this weight loss plan, the Net Carbohydrates have been kept at 5 grams or less for each meal.

This example also allows the dieter to eat every 3 hours for a total of 6 meals during the course of the day. I would wager that most people reading this section will agree this is more food than they thought a person could consume daily and still lose weight.

PROTEIN-gr	CARB-gr	FAT-gr	MEAL DESCRIPTION
Ultra-Low Carb Weight Loss Meal Plan for 150 lb Individual			
8	10 (3)	5	I slice Low Carb Bread, 2 Bacon slices, 1 slice Cheese
14	8 (4)	17	1 Egg, 1 Slice Cheese, 1 Oz Almonds
48	6 (4)	2	Low Carb Protein Shake-Large
32	10 (4)	12	Chicken Salad w/ Low-Carb Tortilla
24	3 (2)	1	Low Carb Protein Shake-Small
30	6 (3)	3	1/2 Grilled Chicken Breast & 1/2 cup Broccoli

Protein-gr	Carb-gr	Fat-gr	TOTAL
156	43	40	CALORIES
Protein-cal	Carb-cal	Fat-cal	CONSUMED
624	172	360	1156
% of Cal.	% of Cal.	% of Cal.	
53.98%	14.88%	31.14%	100.00%

Note- Net Carbohydrates are shown in parenthesis.

This concept brings us back to the opening paragraph of this chapter. Most people who don't feel they are eating very much but still seem to gain weight are probably consuming far more empty calories than they realize.

Consider this example: A handful of store shelf snack crackers may not be very filling, but a typical serving comprises approximately 38 carbohydrates *(ALL of them Net Carbs)*. This snack will also contain 14 grams of fat and less than 6 grams of protein. Total calories in this case will easily add up to over 300 calories. In other words, the amount of carbohydrates found in this single snack food is almost equal to the total carbohydrates consumed in ALL SIX of the meals described in the above example!

Take a moment and let this point sink in. The empty calories and dense carbohydrate concentrations found in most modern processed foods are a major cause of the growing obesity problem we see in the world today.

Losing weight does not necessarily mean eating less. It means eating smarter. People following this kind of meal plan often remark that they can't eat all the food they are allowed to. Being allowed to eat 6 times per day is actually sometimes too much. Weight loss of 3 pounds per week is not uncommon in these cases.

Do not forget the point we made earlier about weight loss goals. Scales are almost useless when it comes to evaluating body composition. The mirror is the most accurate way to determine your proper bodyweight.

This fact exists because a muscular 5'6" individual may weigh 160 pounds, while a soft and flabby person of the same height may only weigh 150 pounds.

Despite this fact, we need a rough idea of what our ideal bodyweight should be when first starting a diet program. Scales do at least offer a general idea of where we stand in terms of estimating weight loss needs. In other words, your bathroom scales will get you in the right ball-park—but the mirror allows you to hit a home run.

I should also take a moment to emphasize another important point. People following a low carbohydrate diet should be mindful to drink plenty of water and remain hydrated. Reduced carbohydrate consumption and subsequent body fat metabolism increases the normal daily requirements for water.

When following a diet such as this, lemon water, unsweetened ice tea, and flavored drinks sweetened with either Stevia or Sucralose are great alternatives for those who desire some variety from plain water. Stay hydrated when following any low carbohydrate diet for weight loss.

When thinking about using an ultra-low carbohydrate meal plan, the goal is to eat primarily high protein, high fiber, and low Glycemic Index carbohydrate foods.

Below is a list that will help you make the right choices:

• •

Good Choices:

Canadian Bacon, Chicken Breast, Cottage Cheese, Eggs, Egg Whites, Fish, Lean Beef, Lean Hamburger Patties, Hard Cheeses, London Broil, Low Carb Breads, Low Carb Protein Powders, Shrimp, Sugar Free Jello®, Top Round Steak, Turkey Breast ,Whey Protein Isolates

Almonds, Cashews, Natural Peanut Butter, Peanuts, Sunflower Seeds, Toasted Soybeans, Walnuts

Asparagus, Black Beans, Broccoli, Cabbage, Celery, Green Beans, Green Peppers, Lettuce, Lima Beans, Onions, Pickles, Red Peppers, Sauerkraut, Spinach

• •

Avoid These Foods except on Cheat Days
(Once Every 14 Days):

Breaded Meats, Deep Fried Foods, Mass-Building Protein Powder Mixes, Non-Lean Beef, Sausage, Side Bacon

Added Sugars, Bread, Cakes, Cereal, Cookies, Crackers, Doughnuts, Granola Bars, Pasta, Potato Chips, Pretzels, Rice, Rolls, Wraps
Beets, Carrots, French Fries, Potatoes, Squash, Sweet Potatoes

Fruit Juice, Ice Cream, Milk, Sweetened Sodas, Yogurt

• •

If you are ever in doubt, today's food labeling requirements make it easy to assess a food's suitability for a low carbohydrate diet.

I have never seen a situation where an ultra-low carbohydrate diet and training routine as described in this book has failed to help a person lose unwanted pounds. The only exception may be those very, very rare individuals with a diagnosed medical condition of the thyroid, adrenals, or hormone systems that creates a unique health situation. However, such medical conditions are extremely rare and only affect an estimated 0.25% of the population. The other 99.75% of us have no excuse.

The most challenging thing for most people is consistency. It only takes some hectic days and a few just-this-one-time trips to a fast food drive-through to totally derail a healthy diet plan.

Stay with it!

Diet Adjustment after Weight Loss

Once a person has lost a desired amount of weight and body fat following an ultra-low carbohydrate diet, what do you do next?

The first response to that question is easy. Do NOT return to your original eating habits that caused you to get overweight and out of shape in the first place.

Too often people think they can diet long enough to lose excess pounds, and then when the weight is lost they feel they can return to their original habits and maintain the new lowered weight. This is flawed thinking.

If the original eating habits were truly a maintenance level, then excess weight would never have been accumulated in the first place. For the person who has lost weight on an ultra-low carbohydrate diet, they must slowly and carefully begin to reintroduce quality carbohydrates into their meals. In a sense, the serious dieter will work backwards through the last few sections regarding weight loss.

After completing an ultra-low carbohydrate diet and reaching a desired body size, the serious dieter will move towards a reduced calorie diet like that we discussed in the previous section dealing with standard weight loss.

Most likely the ideal amount of carbohydrates needed for ongoing weight maintenance will end up being slightly less than our original calculated formula of:

Carbs/day (grams) = Lean Body Weight (lbs) x 1.5/lb

Example: For a person with a lean body weight of 150 lbs
Daily Carbs needed = 150 lbs x 1.5g/lb = 225 grams

With a little trial and error over subsequent weeks, you will find the right amount of quality carbohydrates and frequency of cheat days that allow you to maintain your new lowered body composition.

We are all different. Each of us has inherited different genetics that determine the ease (or difficulty) with which we lose excess body fat. Regardless of our individual differences, the principle for weight loss remains the same.

Be sure to consume the ideal amount of protein and dietary fats for your desired bodyweight. Make adjustments to your carbohydrate consumption and activity levels to lose excess fat. If you remember this basic principle, you will always be on the right track.

In the final analysis, knowing what to do is only half the battle. It is actually doing what you know to be right that is the key to successful results.

In this section, I have used the term "Cheat Days" several times as they relate to weight loss. It is now time to learn how these special days are used to make dietary and lifestyle changes less dramatic.

Cheat Days

The body is a machine highly capable of adaption. This ability to adapt is usually a wonderful thing. In fact, the ability to adapt is why exercise and training are effective in the first place. By pushing the body to perform at a higher level than it is accustomed to, it will adapt to that increased workload in the form of stronger bones and muscles, increased bone density, higher endurance, and better flexibility.

But the body's ability to adapt can also work against us sometimes. When we go on any kind of diet that severely reduces calories for an amount of time, the body thinks it may forever be forced to work with a lower level of caloric intake.

What does the body do at this point? It takes steps to prevent the possibility of what it fears may be impending starvation. The body's natural preservation programming starts to slow down the metabolism. This can create a vicious cycle for dieters who unknowingly go on crash diets to try to lose weight. With the drastic reduction of calories, the metabolism starts to slow down in response. The individual gets frustrated that he can no longer lose weight and decides to cut calories even more. Again the body reacts by slowing the metabolism.

This cycle becomes a losing proposition for the dieter, as eventually the only way to overcome the body's preservation mechanism of slowing the metabolism is to almost starve one's self. Yes, a near starvation diet will lead to weight loss, but it also leads to a loss of muscle tissue (as we learned earlier, lean muscle helps control basal metabolism), as well as other nutritional deficiencies. Furthermore, a climate is created where the individual will more easily gain weight again after they quit starving themselves since their metabolism has been wrecked.

You may know or even have personal experience with "Yo-Yo" dieters. The term Yo-Yo dieting refers to people who are able to lose weight on a diet, but then quickly regain all the weight they lost after they go off the diet. In fact, many times not only do the people regain the weight they lost, they actually end up gaining more.

For the most part, diets do not work. This may sound like a controversial statement, but I will explain.

A "diet" is not the same thing as making long term dietary changes. Many people think of a diet as something they do for a short period of time to lose unwanted pounds, with the idea that once those pounds are lost they can resume their old eating habits and maintain themselves at the new lower weight.

99% of the time, this does not work. Think about it. If this idea was logical and scientifically sound, the extra weight would never have been gained in the first place. The individual would have remained at the same weight to begin with.

The only way to have long term weight control is to make lasting lifestyle changes to your diet. The process we described above for calculating protein, fat, and carbohydrate requirements for your body is the framework upon which your typical daily dieting should be based.

This sounds great in theory you say, but, "What about those great cookies my sister bakes?" "What about that World Famous Key Lime Pie when I visit Key West Florida?"

I agree. A professional athlete in training for a major competition may have to make extreme sacrifices for a stretch of time, but not we normal people just trying to stay in shape. We can still enjoy the culinary pleasures of life by utilizing cheat days in an intelligently planned way.

A cheat day is essentially a day where you allow yourself to enjoy those white chocolate macadamia cookies or those rich walnut brownies. As just discussed, if we reduce our calories continuously for a long stretch of time, our body naturally begins to slow down our metabolism. For weight control, this is an undesirable condition. We want to keep our metabolism at a healthy level.

By having a cheat day once every 7 or 14 days, we "surprise" the body by boosting the total calories for a day. Then immediately the next day we are back to our normal clean eating routine for the next week or two (with no more cheating!).

This sporadic alteration to our calorie consumption prevents the body from adapting to a perceived permanent caloric reduction. Likewise a few hundred more calories 2–4 times per month are not enough added calories to seriously hamper your weight control goals.

There are some things to keep in mind when it comes to cheat days. They are not an excuse to binge eat everything in sight and eat until you are literally sick. A cheat day is simply a strategically used day you can look forward to for enjoying your favorite treats in life and not feeling as though your healthy lifestyle is depriving you in any way. The cheat day not only lets you still enjoy your favorite "bad foods", but also serves the beneficial purpose of tricking your metabolism so that it does not begin to downshift on you.

We said that a cheat day is used once every 7 or 14 days. How do you determine how often you can have a cheat day?

As with most things in life, common sense provides the right answer. If you are not seriously overweight or are within a few pounds of your desired size, then you can probably afford one cheat day per week. By comparison, if you are working hard to lose 10, 15, 20 pounds or more, then you should probably limit yourself to a cheat day every 14 days.

I will relate my own personal experiences to you. I worked my way through college in the 1980s as a cook in several restaurants. One of the nicer summer jobs I worked back then also required me to attend a chef school. The result is that I have always done most of the cooking in our home (a fact that makes my wife very happy).

Fast forward to today. We have friends over every other Saturday night for movies and dinner. I usually try a new recipe for both dinner and dessert each time we are together. Most of the time, I eat following the guidelines and examples described in this book, but I treat these Saturday get-togethers as my 14 day cheat day.

There was a time when that was the only cheat day I could allow myself, as I was still trying to lose substantial weight. These days, my weight remains in the 203–210 pound range. Because I am able to remain in this relatively narrow bodyweight bracket, I am now able to have a cheat day every 7 days.

My wife enjoys the pizza I make with homemade dough using high gluten flour and an old authentic Italian recipe, so we sometimes have that once a week or every other week. So these days, being at my desired body size, I can afford one cheat day per week. If I catch my weight creeping upwards, I first reduce my cheat days before making any other dietary changes to determine where I'm really at. Often times this is enough to get me back on track.

One more comment about cheat days. At no time should they become more frequent than once every 7 days. If you begin to make a habit of eating cookies, cakes, pizzas, and key lime pies every day of the week (or even every other day) they are no longer strategically planned cheat days—they simply become bad eating habits.

Gaining Weight Diet Modifications

If you happened to just finish reading the previous sections on losing weight, then you probably already figured out what you need to do to gain weight.

Do the exact opposite of what we discussed above. Instead of cutting 500 carbohydrate calories or so per day, you will want to INCREASE the amount of carbohydrates you consume. The preferred foods to achieve this include both complex and starchy carbohydrates such as oats, breads, pasta, potatoes, rice and the like.

Since weight control is not the critical concern for people wishing to gain weight, the timing of eating increased carbohydrates around periods of physical activity is not as important. Those wishing to gain weight can spread the consumption of these extra carbs evenly though out the day.

Sample Recipes

Many times when people think about healthy eating, they fear they will be condemned to a life of bland, tasteless, boring food. Such is not the case. Many of us grew up accustomed to styles of cooking that rely heavily on fats and salt for flavoring. Many good old "country-style" recipes need loads of butter and salt to taste good. Over the last few decades in America, foreign and exotic foods that don't depend on butter and salt for their flavor have become more commonplace across the country.

There are several good books available that offer great tasting recipes for those trying to clean up their eating habits. You will find a few of these titles listed in the Suggested Reading appendix at the end of this book. For now, I want to offer just a few recipes that demonstrate how flavorful healthy cooking can be.

Tiger Tear – Thai Beef Salad

One of my best friends owned an award-winning Thai restaurant in South Florida. For many years, my wife and I visited his place every Thursday night for our weekly date night. He always promised me if he decided to return to Thailand, he would teach us how to prepare our favorite dishes. A few years ago my friend did indeed move back to Asia, but we still keep in contact to this day. I want to thank Paul Triam for this beef salad recipe. No doubt, you will thank him too after you taste it.

Ingredients:

9 oz Top Round or Flank Steak *(trimmed lean)*

1/2 Onion *(thinly sliced)*

1/2 Red Bell Pepper *(thinly sliced)*

1 PF Cilantro *(chopped)*

1/2 t Sugar *

1 T Fish Sauce

1 T Lemon Juice

2 T Water

1 t Cayenne Pepper

1 t Spanish Paprika

1/4 HD Lettuce

Directions:

1. Thinly slice **Steak** into strips *(2 inches long x 1/4" wide)*.
2. Grill meat and rinse off the char.
3. Place grilled meat in a medium bowl.
4. Add the sliced **Onion, Red Pepper** and **Cilantro** to bowl.
5. Add 1/2 Teaspoon **Sugar** to bowl.
6. Add 1 Tablespoon **Fish Sauce** to bowl.
7. Add 1 Tablespoon of **Vinegar** and 2 Tablespoons of **Water** to bowl.
8. Add 1 Tablespoon **Lemon Juice**.
9. Mix by hand.
10. Add 1 Teaspoon each of **Paprika** and **Cayenne Pepper** to mixture and stir gently to blend.
11. *Optional – Add chopped Thai Peppers if extra-hot is desired.*
12. Chop 1/4 head of iceberg **Lettuce**.
14. Add mixture to chopped lettuce.

Legend:

t=teaspoon   T=Tablespoon   HD=Head   PF=Palmful

Makes 2 servings

Each serving: Protein-32 gr.   Carbs-22 gr.   Fat-6 gr.

* Ultra Low Carb dieters can substitute a Sucralose or Stevia sweetener for the sugar.

Jamaican Jerk Chicken Tossed Salad

Since many people like salads with grilled chicken, I have included this recipe that has more flavor than you will find in most restaurant offerings. This recipe features an oven-baked chicken breast seasoned with hot and spicy Jamaican Jerk seasoning. This is also a fast and easy recipe to prepare.

Ingredients:

8 oz   Boneless Skinless Chicken Breast

1-2 T   Walkerswood Jamaican Jerk Seasoning® *(to taste)*

3 C   Tossed Salad Blend

2 T   Salad Dressing *(Catalina or Parmesan recommended)*

1/4 C   Mexican style mixed Cheese Blend *(shredded)*

Sp   Salad Supreme Seasoning® *(McCormick's brand)*

Sp   Black Pepper

Directions:

1. Slice **Chicken Breast** into 4 equal sized pieces.
2. Rub & cover the chicken breast pieces with **Jerk Seasoning.**
3. Bake or Broil Chicken at 375 degrees for 25-30 minutes.
4. Turn chicken several times to ensure even cooking.
5. Remove chicken from oven and allow it to cool slightly.
6. Meanwhile, toss **Salad Blend**, **Dressing** and **Cheese**.
7. Slice cooked chicken into smaller pieces and toss into salad.
8. Sprinkle with **Salad Supreme** and **Black Pepper** to taste.

Legend:

oz=Ounces   T=Tablespoon   Sp=Sprinkle   C=Cups

Makes 2 servings

Each serving: Protein-28 gr.   Carbs-12 gr.   Fat-13 gr.

This Chapter in Summary

✦ Eat for the body you want, not the body you have.

✦ Use the formulas below to calculate the correct amount of Protein, Fat, and Carbohydrates needed to feed your desired bodyweight.

✦ Determine Daily Protein Requirements (grams) as Desired Bodyweight (lbs) x 1.0

✦ Determine Daily Fat Requirements (grams) as Desired Bodyweight (lbs) x 0.2

✦ Determine the base level of Daily Carbohydrates needed (grams) as Desired Bodyweight lbs) x 1.5

✦ Eat 4–6 small meals with protein, fats, and carbohydrates consumed each meal.

✦ Protein and fat consumption should always remain fairly constant based on your desired lean bodyweight goals.

✦ Limit consumption of saturated fats while totally avoiding trans-fats.

✦ Eat more carbohydrates in the 2–3 hours before and after times of peak physical activity. Eat fewer carbohydrates during times of less activity or close to bedtime.

✦ Only make adjustments to carbohydrates consumed when attempting to either lose or gain weight.

✦ When cutting carbohydrates for weight loss, you should reduce the simple sugars first. Many people find that simply eliminating empty calories like donuts, cakes, candy, and other sugar-loaded sweets are enough to help them lose their unwanted pounds.

✦ Those with a history of difficulty losing weight and/or with substantial body fat may need to consider an ultra-low carbohydrate diet.

Such a diet consists of only 30–50 total carbohydrates per day. The carbohydrates consumed with this kind of meal plan must all be complex and low Glycemic Index foods. Optimum weight loss results can be achieved by insuring no more than 5 Net Carbohydrates are consumed at each meal.

✦ Protein shakes are an excellent way to supplement your meal plan. Low carbohydrate protein shakes make it easier to get the protein you need while keeping overall calories down. When shopping for a quality protein powder, look for a product that is easily mixable and contains enzymes like lactase to aid in digestion. Whey protein in the form of whey protein isolates have been shown to be especially beneficial for older individuals.

✦ Stay hydrated by drinking approximately 8 ounces of water daily. Exact hydration condition can be determined by urine color and urination frequency.

✦ Home distilling water for drinking purposes is affordable and offers many advantages.

✦ Once every 7 or 14 days, have a Cheat Day to enjoy your favorite treats and avoid feeling deprived while at the same time preventing the metabolism from going into adaptive slowdown when dieting.

✦ The mirror is a much better tool than scales for determining your weight loss needs. Muscle tissue, water weight, and fat all have different densities. Looking only at a total weight number on a scale gives no accurate information in terms of your body's actual composition. Two people can be the exact same height and bodyweight, but they will look quite differently if one is all muscle and the other is mostly fat.

Chapter Four

The Nuts and Bolts of Weight Training & Cardio

Sets, Reps, Intensity, and
Other Important Concepts

In the introductory chapter of this book, I explained that my goal was not to write an all-encompassing, massive text that would cover every theory known to man about fitness and exercise. Instead it was stressed that our aim was to get the best bang for the buck and look to years of historical success to find the best diet and exercise advice which has been proven time and again to yield real results. Taking into consideration the special issues that face an aging human machine, we need to adapt these proven techniques to our needs over the age of 40.

In this chapter I will cover some important terminology regarding exercise, discuss selecting a gym, answer the most common questions people usually have about weight resistance training, and look at a number of other important concepts.

Why Weight Resistance Training?

Weight training may be the closest thing we have to an anti-aging miracle. This may sound like a grand statement, but I am not alone in this belief. Do a simple search on the Internet and you will find thousands of hits for "weight training," "anti-aging," and "strength training" in various combinations.

Weight training is a fantastic method of fighting the aging process. As we discussed earlier, muscle loss normally occurs at a rate of 4% every 10 years in adults, increasing to 10% for those over 50. By 60 years of age some people will have lost 30% of their original muscle mass. By continuing to train with weights, it is possible to significantly slow this atrophy process. This means remaining stronger, more mobile, and fitter as you age.

Despite the established benefits of weight training, it seems the older we get the fewer of us continue to carry out any form of regular exercise. Estimates reveal only 6% of those over age 65 exercise regularly and only 4% of those over 75 pursue any form of regular physical activity.

As demonstrated in the nursing home research studies we discussed earlier, conducting light weight training regimens three times per week can have a massive effect on an individual's strength, balance, mobility, flexibility, and coordination, as well as overall health.

Why Cardiovascular Exercise Alone is Not Enough

Cardiovascular exercise in the form of brisk walking, running, elliptical machine, treadmill, biking, or other form of exercise is extremely beneficial. In fact, cardiovascular training plays an important part in the regimen we will be describing in this book. But cardiovascular exercise alone, in the form of jogging for example, is not the optimum method for overall conditioning or even weight loss.

Some people rely solely on running as a means to control weight and stay in good shape. Running certainly benefits the lungs, heart, and circulatory system. Runners usually have strong legs as well. But running does very little to strengthen the upper half of the body. Additionally, in the absence of any muscle tissue building exercise to increase muscle mass and subsequently boost the metabolism, runners often find themselves needing to increase the distances or speeds they run to continue weight control.

Some people that rely only on running for exercise acquire a drawn look with narrow shoulders, thin arms, and an almost unhealthy appearance. This look is usually only seen in those relying exclusively on diet and running for exercise and weight control, but it does serve to demonstrate that cardio alone is not the answer for overall fitness goals.

Why Diet Alone is Not Enough

Some people rely solely on diet as a means to control body weight. Once again we must stress that when a person severely cuts calories to lose weight in the absence of any kind of muscle toning exercise, they face a potential problem with muscle atrophy and a slowing metabolism. This slowing metabolism causes the individual to further cut calories if they desire to keep their weight low.

Another problem with dieting as the solitary means of controlling weight is a phenomenon often referred to as becoming a "skinny fat person." What is a skinny fat person? The best answer to this question is a simple example: Have you ever seen a paparazzi photograph of a famous celebrity who you thought was lean, fit, and trim when you saw them in clothing, but in candid beach photos they appear saggy and baggy despite being thin?

This is commonly seen in fashion models and aging celebrities (male and female) who are desperate to remain slim, but do so only through strict dieting while apparently eschewing any form of serious resistance exercise. What results is loose sagging skin hanging over a skeletal frame with virtually no muscular shape but just a layer of cellulite or fat under the skin. Men may exhibit belly fat and "man boobs" while women will possess fat on the back of the legs and a saggy look around the knees and triceps area of the arms. A body composition test would reveal these people to have a higher percentage of body fat than muscle despite being slim or skinny. If you think of some famous movie starlets or aging male singers that are often captured in the pages of notable tabloid magazines, you probably know exactly what "skinny fat" is.

Needless to say, this is not the type of fitness and conditioning we are looking to achieve. It is the three-part combination of diet + weight resistance training + cardiovascular exercise that will give you the results you desire.

How Often Do I Need To Exercise?

Numerous TV ads will tell you that they can help you lose weight and get in shape with no exercise, no change to your normal routine, and no change in your current eating habits.

I will say this one time. These companies are lying to 99% of you.

Very rare are the people so blessed with perfect genetics that they can go through life eating everything they want and only taking an occasional walk or game of golf and stay firm, trim, and fit as they age. In fact, if you were among this rare group of genetically gifted people, there is a strong chance you would not even be reading this book right now.

Most of us have to make some basic lifestyle changes that enable us to fight back against the forces of time as we pass the age of 40.

If by now you are convinced that most of the fancy gimmicks and empty promises sold on TV are a lie just to take your money and make somebody else rich, you are probably thinking to yourself, "Okay, I realize there is no effortless way to stay in shape, so how many days a week am I really looking at here?"

The answer is three days per week.

Three days per week you will be doing some form of weight resistance and cardio training. Obviously this will be combined with the daily application of dietary principles discussed in the previous chapter.

Time wise you will be looking at 30–45 minutes of weight training and 30–45 minutes of cardio training each session. This equates to a total of 60–90 minutes of structured exercise three times per week.

Another way of looking at this is 2.7% of your total time each week. Ideally we would like those days to be spread out across the week to allow time for recovery. Thus it would be better to work out every other day as compared to exercising three days in a row, then resting for four days.

I don't know about you, but I confess I probably waste 3–5 hours per week surfing the Internet or watching some bad TV shows. So the time can be found if you are serious about your health.

Where Should I Workout?

People will exercise most effectively where they feel most comfortable. With this thought in mind, I strongly urge joining a gym or fitness center of some kind. Why do I make this recommendation? There are a number of reasons:

- Gyms offer a variety of equipment almost impossible to duplicate at home unless you have lots of square footage and money to spare.

- Studies show most people are more motivated if they treat the trip to the gym as a planned activity instead of just something they squeeze in while hanging around the house.

- There are often distractions around the home that interfere with exercise discipline and consistency.

- Social relationships are sometimes more scarce as we get older. The gym environment offers an opportunity to meet other people, exercise together, and learn new techniques.

- Commercial gym facilities, especially those associated with hospitals, can offer quick medical response if needed.

I have had memberships at a number of different types of facilities over the years. I have trained at YMCAs, community activity centers, hardcore gyms populated with bodybuilding competitors, modern commercial franchised gyms like LA Fitness, Bally, and Golds. Lastly I have trained at fitness centers affiliated with regional hospitals.

We are all different in our tastes regarding atmosphere, but I personally prefer the hospital gyms over all others now that I am in my 50s. Many commercially franchised gyms tend to cater to younger clientele. This often results in overcrowding and loud music that borders on feeling more like a night club than a gym. This may actually be desirable for some older folks who like the idea of surrounding themselves with a younger crowd while exercising to hip-hop, techno, salsa, and rap music blasting at 110 decibels. That is not the case for me, or most older people I have met.

My experience has been that fitness centers associated with hospitals have smaller crowds, an older clientele, quieter atmospheres, and they offer all the best equipment. Often time these gyms are also less expensive.

Hospital fitness centers are more geared towards using the gym facilities for their physical therapy and rehabilitation patients. Outside members are an added bonus to their revenue stream, but not their primary focus. As a result, they do not mass market and advertise their facilities to the public at large to generate high traffic and massive membership volume.

All in all, I feel this makes for a more pleasant training experience for the majority of older individuals.

Most likely, you will desire to visit a number of facilities in your area to see which gym best suits your personal tastes.

Unless you are willing to spend the money to set up a fully-equipped gym in your home, I again emphasize that I feel joining a gym is your optimum choice for exercise location. However, it is understood there are individuals who may be in a situation where this is not an option.

You can exercise at home and still gain considerable benefit with only a small investment in some basic equipment. Following the chapters detailing our recommended exercise regimens, you will find a chapter dedicated to a home-based routine. In that chapter, we will modify our gym-based workout regimen for use at home utilizing dumbbells along with a few other pieces of affordable gear.

What Should I Wear When Exercising?

The best answer to this question is to wear whatever is comfortable.

Certainly your choice of workout clothing will vary based on climate, but as a rule you should dress in such a way that you have freedom of movement. Additionally you should not be excessively hot or cold.

Plastic sweat suits or other similar clothing that claim to aid in weight loss are discouraged. These types of outfits do virtually

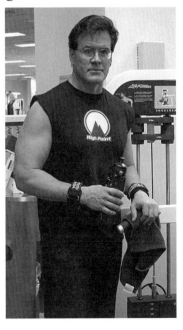

(Photo 4.1) Sweat pants and a large, loose t-shirt allow freedom of motion and prove a great choice for exercise clothing.

nothing of benefit, but can cause excess water loss, dehydration, and heat exhaustion.

Personally, my favorite exercise clothing consists of sweat pants and sleeveless t-shirts. Both items are 100% cotton. The long sweat pants help keep my legs warm (but not too hot) and thus soothe any minor knee pains. The sleeveless t-shirt allows free unrestricted motion of my arms for chest, shoulder, back, bicep, and triceps exercises.

How Much Weight Should I Lift?

This is a common question, but the answer is actually very simple. Do not worry about some preconceived idea of how much weight you should be using for exercise, your body will tell you the proper amount to use.

Over the last half century, much research has been done to determine the optimum number of repetitions of an exercise needed to attain a certain goal. A repetition is a single performance of an exercise. For example, if you were asked to do 10 sit-ups, that would be called 10 repetitions.

In exercise jargon, the word repetition is often abbreviated to "reps."

Without boring you with tons of references and study results, I will tell you that general consensus is as follows:

- 4–6 repetitions are best suited for building maximum power.

- 6–8 repetitions are good for building strength and size.

- 8–12 repetitions combine both size and strength gains with some endurance benefit.

- 15–20+ repetitions are best for endurance and toning.

These guidelines are approximate ranges that have been shown over time to be best suited for reaching specific goals. Obviously, some overlap and genetic variation between individuals will cause different people to see varied results, but this general guide holds true for most people.

Basically, if you are lifting heavy weights for fewer than 6 repetitions you will be developing brute strength. Conversely, if you lift a lighter weight 15 times or more, you will develop endurance and help tone the muscle with less increase in strength or fiber size.

You will find professional bodybuilders vary their routines throughout the year between heavy weight/low repetitions and medium weight/moderate repetitions so they can fully develop all their muscle fibers in different ways. But for non-professional athletes such as ourselves, we need not worry about getting this specialized.

How does this repetition information apply to those of us looking for the most effective way to train past 40? We should keep two factors in mind:

- With age, we must be more careful to protect joints, cartilage, and tendons.

- As explained earlier, we lose Fast Twitch muscle fibers much more quickly than Slow Twitch fibers as we age. Fast Twitch fibers, you will recall, are responsible for strength, speed, and much of your muscle mass that affects your Basal Metabolic Rate.

Older people may not have any problem taking long, slow walks around the neighborhood, but activities that require strength and speed such as flipping mattresses or getting up from a couch become more difficult with age.

Taking both of these factors into consideration, it turns out 8–12 repetitions is the "sweet spot" target range for us when designing a weight training program. In fact, we will be incorporating one higher repetition set of 15–20 reps as a warm up set when we begin each new exercise. After that, our working sets will normally be in the 8–12 range.

This examination of repetitions leads us to the answer for our original question of "How Much Weight Should I Lift?" We can now answer that question properly.

The amount of weight you select to lift for each exercise should be enough that you are able to complete 10 repetitions before reaching failure. We define "failure" as the point where you can not perform one more repetition with proper form.

In actual practice this means if the weight is so heavy you can't lift it more than 5–6 times, you are using too much weight. On the other hand, if you zoom right through 12, 13, 14, 15 repetitions and you could still do plenty more, the weight is too light.

Why does this method work for proper weight selection? By using a weight you can lift 10 times before approaching failure, you are not placing too much strain on the supporting structure of the joints and connective tissue as would be the case if you were trying to hoist much heavier poundage for fewer reps. Ten is also the middle of our target range of 8–12 repetitions for optimally adding both strength and lean muscle tissue.

How Fast Should I Be Lifting When Performing Weight Resistance Exercises?

Along with knowing the preferred number of repetitions to perform for deriving the best results from our exercise routine, another thing to be considered is "rep speed." Rep Speed is how quickly we raise and lower the weight when we do each repetition of an exercise.

We need to protect our joints while also targeting the Fast Twitch muscle fibers that fade more quickly as we age. This is best accomplished by using a slight acceleration to the motion when we lift the weight.

I really want to stress an important point here. We are **NOT** talking about jerking the weights or otherwise using a haphazard technique.

Lifting the weights with slight acceleration means you are not just moving in slow motion, but you are actually pushing the weight upwards with a forward motion that is marginally faster than the return motion to the exercise's starting point. Think of opening a heavy door that swings inward. You do not grab the handle and slowly open the door at a constant speed. Instead you give the door a bit of a push forward to overcome inertia.

The reason we want to use this slight acceleration is to help focus more of the muscle stimulation on our Fast Twitch muscle fibers.

Some reference sources will define repetition speed in terms of how quickly you should perform each individual rep. Technically this definition is accurate, but it proves to be very difficult to measure accurately in real practice.

In real world applications, you will find that 10 repetitions of an exercise should take between 20–40 seconds to complete.

You can expect to be on the lower end of this range for exercises like bicep curls, while bigger exercises like leg presses will take longer due to the heavier weights and greater length of travel. Once again, we don't want to be "exploding" or lifting the weights in an excessively fast, jerky manner—but we do want to lift the weight with a slightly accelerated push and lower the weight more slowly.

Always Exercise Using a Full and Natural Range of Motion

In the first chapter of this book we described a common mistake people make when exercising. We used the example of a leg press machine being loaded with far too much weight and then only moved a few inches. As we explained, this error would offer very little benefit to the leg muscles, but would impose great stress and potential injury to the knee joint. This kind of mistake is something I see every single time I go to a gym.

When we perform weight resistance training, we need to keep two principles in mind:

- You should lift the weight through a full range of motion.

- You should lift the weight following the natural path of your body's motion.

As we age, it is natural for our joints to change both their range of movement and also the angles at which they operate. Additionally, there are commonly recognized differences in male and female anatomy that slightly alter the natural range of motion and angles that our bodies operate.

Refer to the comparative anatomical image in Photo 4.2.

We see a male and female anatomy standing totally relaxed with their arms hanging by their side. You will notice the man's elbows flare out slightly. The shoulders and arms have tendency to roll forwards keeping the elbows further out to the sides while causing the hands to acquire a slight palms-down position.

With the woman's anatomy, you will notice the elbows fall more inwards towards the body, causing the wrists to flare out wider. The lower arm tends to have a more palms-up position.

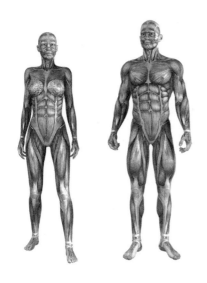

(Photo 4.2) Standing relaxed and natural, the subtle yet fundamental differences in male and female anatomy in terms of natural joint movement are easily visible.

This is not 100% universal, but it is an anatomical variance seen between men and women 85–90% of the time. The differences in shoulder width, back muscle size, breast size, and muscle dominance are largely the cause of this phenomenon. In the next picture, two people were asked to perform a simple curl with dumbbells. You can see the different path and range of motion naturally preferred by each subject. Their natural preference reflects the observations made above.

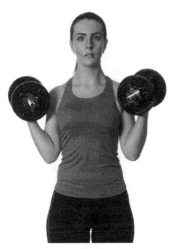
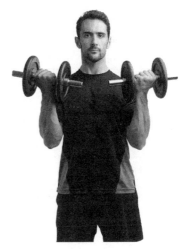

(Photo 4.3) Notice how the basic difference in natural arm position causes each individual to naturally follow a different path and range of motion when performing a bicep curl with dumbbells.

As we will learn, there are advantages to using different exercises to work our muscles completely and from all angles. There is also benefit to using different hand positions with the same exercise to change portions of the muscle being targeted.

But despite this, we must always remember that our goal is to work the muscles as much as possible while minimizing unnatural motion or torque on our joints and other connective tissue. Along with the idea of a natural range of motion, we are also stressing the importance of a full range of motion.

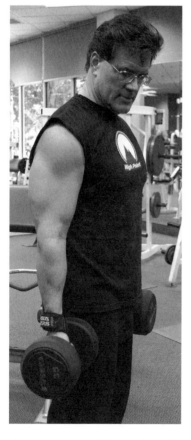
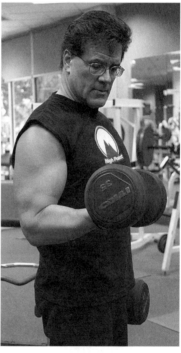

(Photo 4.4) Correct execution of a biceps curl using dumbbells. Notice the elbows remain at the sides of the body. The weights begin in the full down position. The weight is curled upwards as far as possible using the bicep muscle without changing the position of the elbow.

This again alludes to the leg press example we gave earlier. You should always be performing an exercise through a full range of motion.

Do **NOT** perform small partial movements. Using the biceps curl as an example, the photos over these three pages show both correct and incorrect technique for this exercise.

Throughout this book, while describing and demonstrating exercises, I will repeatedly stress the importance of this important principle. I will also provide things to look out for specific to each motion.

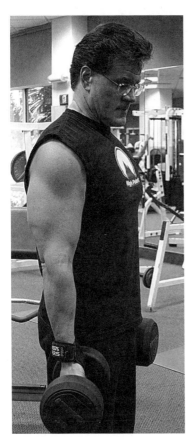
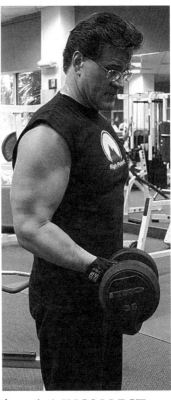

(Photo 4.5) INCORRECT execution of a biceps curl using dumbbells. Notice the arm is barely moving much at all between the start and finish positions.

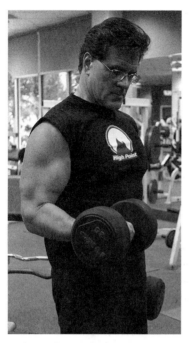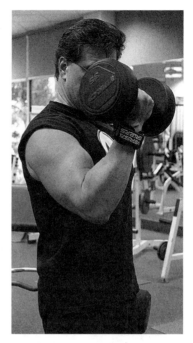

(Photo 4.6) INCORRECT execution of a biceps curl using dumbbells. Notice the arm is always bent at a 90 degree angle at the elbow. The elbow has moved away from the side of the body and the weight is near the chin. Since the arm is not bending at the elbow, the biceps muscle of the frontal arm is doing virtually no work. The major lifting power is being provided by the frontal deltoids in this example of bad technique.

✦ Important Principle ✦

Always Use a Full And Natural Range of Motion When Performing Weight Resistance Exercises.

Protect Your Back with Proper Posture When Lifting Weights

Far too many people over the age of 40 (and even younger actually) have lower back problems. One very common cause of these back problems is the habit of bending at the waist to lift heavy objects.

In its natural anatomically strong position, the spinal column forms a gentle S-shape (Photo 4.7).

The spinal column is flexible by nature of its design. Essentially, the spine is a series of 33 vertebrae stacked on top of each other with each section of bone being separated and cushioned by a fibrocartilage disc (Photo 4.8).

This construction allows you to bend, twist, stretch, arch, and perform an almost infinite number of combined motions in your everyday life.

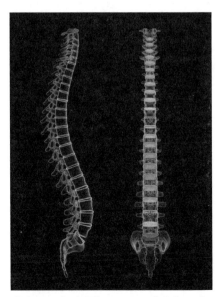

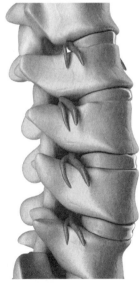

(Photo 4.7) The natural S-bend shape of the spinal column.

(Photo 4.8) Vertebrae and Discs of the Human Spine.

But like any machine, the human body is still at the mercy of the laws of gravity, physics, and leverage.

Why does bent-over lifting often damage human backs with time? When a heavy object is lifted while maintaining the back in its natural S-bend arch, the distribution of force is fairly equally applied across all the surface area of the intervertebral discs. By comparison, once an individual bends over, they are effectively applying increased pressure on a leading edge of those vertebrae that are involved in the bending motion. Much of this imbalanced force distribution occurs in the lumbar region of the lower back.

Discs are designed with a tough outer coating and a softer jelly-like inner material. Whiles disc don't literally "slip out of place," they can be damaged. Under excessive pressure, the disc can bulge out beyond its normal position and the outer casing can tear or rupture. This is called a herniated disc.

Bending forward with a rounded back (bending forward from the waist) is more risky than bending forward with a straight neutral back (pivoting forward from the hips). Lifting with a rounded back creates excessive compression at the front of the disc and more pressure at the back of the disc. The disc's contents are essentially forced backward under what can be thought of as hydraulic pressure.

Intuitively this makes a lot of sense when you think about it. You can mentally envision how the vertebrae of your lower back must be sitting "on edge" when you are in a bent over, rounded back position. Now, add a heavy weight that may be held out in front of you. The law of leverage multiplies the effective force being applied to those bent discs.

Think of this simple analogy. Pretend you have a small, flat piece of metal that must be bent. If you lay it flat on the table, no matter how much downwards pressure you apply, the metal does not bend. It is supported equally by the table beneath it.

If you lift one side of the metal off the table and press downwards, it will only be supported by a leading edge. Now apply downwards pressure, and the metal will bend in the middle close to where it rests on the table. Applying force to an equally balanced object is much different than applying the same force to an imbalanced object that is under a leveraged position.

✦ Important Principle ✦

It is best to maintain a straight, neutral back position when lifting heavy weights.

Pivot forward from the hips when lifting. Do not bend forward with a rounded back position when lifting moderate to heavy weights.

Many times in the pages to follow, I will keep repeating and stressing the importance of proper back position when lifting weights.

In the meantime, in everyday life, here are some useful guidelines to remember when lifting.

- Squat down using legs while maintaining a straight back position.

- Lift and hold items close to your body so as to maintain a good center of gravity.

- Keep feet approximately shoulder-width apart.

- Keep stomach muscles tight

- Lift with your legs, not your back.

- Do not twist or rotate while carrying a heavy weight. If you must change direction, stop and change your position with small steps first.

- Keep the neck straight and eyes forward when lifting heavy items.

I know it may seem as though I beat this topic to death, but I feel it is very important. Good lower back health is a blessing.

Ask anybody who suffers from continual back pain or weakness how it adversely affects their quality of life. You will soon appreciate the importance of having a pain-free back that allows you to participate in your favorite activities without restrictions.

How Much Rest Should I Take Between Working Sets?

The amount of rest needed between working sets will vary slightly depending on the size of the muscle group being exercised. Lifting heavier weights with the legs will be more tiring than lifting lighter weights with your arms.

You will find that it will take a little longer for your breathing to return to normal after a set of leg presses as compared to a set of bicep curls. With this fact in mind, you should be resting in the range of 30–90 seconds depending on if you are working a small or large muscle group.

Is There A Rule For Breathing When Lifting Weights?

The only hard and fast rule regarding breathing is to **NEVER** hold your breath while exerting yourself or lifting weights.

The reason you don't want to hold your breath while lifting weights, exerting yourself, or bending over to lift an item, is because this action will increase intra-thoracic pressure. Elevated intra-thoracic pressure can increase blood pressure, place extra strain on internal organs, cause dizziness or fainting, and aggravate hernias, to name only a few concerns.

The best way to breathe while lifting weights is to exhale when you are exerting force. Inhale when you are returning to a starting position.

An excellent way to remember this habit is to think of Karate. Have you noticed when Karate masters strike a blow, they shout "Kiai"? The trained habit of yelling this word ensures the individual will be exhaling when they explosively exert their maximum force. If we compare this to lifting weights, you can easily remember that you should be exhaling when you lift the weight, and taking in your next breath as you return the weight to its starting position.

Additionally, when doing exercises for the midsection, it is generally considered wise to exhale during motions where you are shortening your torso and inhale when lengthening the torso.

Think of the common sit ups you probably performed in school. As you sit forward, more internal pressure builds up inside your body's organs as muscles contract and you crunch into a curled position. It would be unwise to inhale at this time, as it would only serve to increase pressure on the diaphragm and thoracic region. Exhaling during the forward motion of the sit up allows for better movement, more comfort, and minimal build up of internal pressures.

Do I Perform These Exercise Routines Year Round?

It is beneficial to take at least one week off from regimented training every 4–6 months. During this time, you may prefer to take longer walks or participate in some other activities such as swimming or bike riding.

As we discussed earlier, the body adapts to repetition. Taking a break from regular training at strategically timed intervals during the year throws our body a small curve ball.

These breaks also allow us to heal from any minor injuries or aches we may have acquired in the previous months. For those still working regular jobs, it is convenient to use vacations as the times to take scheduled training breaks.

How Long to See and Feel Results?

We live in a society where all too often people have come to expect instant gratification and satisfaction. Advances in technology have certainly made these high expectations reasonable in regards to many things like instantly downloading software, or streaming movies to our home HD televisions.

Early man was not much different than our animal counterparts. The majority of our time was spent seeking food, water, and shelter. Perpetuation of the species via reproduction was another driving force.

With the creation of our modern society, we have changed the priorities and principle issues upon which our survival is based. No longer do we spend long hours of each day hunting or farming our own food. Instead, we now work jobs to earn money that in turn is used to purchase the necessities of life (and more). The career path and 9–5 job is the hunting and farming of today for most people in the modern world.

Our human bodies however, still essentially function today as they did thousands of years ago. The human body is highly adaptable to changes in stimulation; however, these adaptations are not instantaneous. For example, if you perform heavy strenuous work on a house project for a week or two, your body is not going to suddenly change its baseline fitness level. Your body is conservative by design and will attempt to deal with any short term changes in diet or activity level using its current structure.

Think about the human body as it is designed to work in nature. It would be illogical for the body to easily add new muscle fiber and increase bone density as a result of the smallest extra effort. This would require hunting or farming for even more food to fuel this newly enhanced body.

When you first start lifting weights, your body is not going to suddenly change its level of protein synthesis and create new muscle fiber for what may only be a temporary situation. During the first few weeks of exercise, your body will try to strengthen existing ligaments, tendons, and muscles to deal with the new demands being placed upon it. The number of existing muscle fibers being recruited may increase as your body tries to get the most out of what it already has.

But let us look down the road eight or ten weeks. If this new demand of physical activity has not relented, your body comes to a realization. It essentially says to itself, "Hmm, this existing body is not going to cut it when it comes to dealing with these new demands. It is time to make some modifications."

It is only then that truly noticeable changes begin to occur—the kind of changes that you see in the mirror or friends and family comment about. Yes, of course you were benefiting from exercise early on, but really noticeable changes in appearance and endurance don't begin until the 12–16 week mark.

Does this fact surprise you? In our instant gratification society where TV infomercials promise a new body in 10 days (deceptive marketing) and drug companies promise a pill to cure every ailment, 12–16 weeks may sound like a long time. But this 3–4 month timeframe is the honest truth.

If you are reading this book, it is a good chance you are over 40 years of age and have been unhappy with your level of fitness for some time. Perhaps you have tried a variety of programs or apparatus in the past, only to be discouraged after 3–4 weeks. Perhaps you gave up. How long ago was that? At our age, we all know time feels to be moving faster and faster every day.

I don't care what any fancy TV commercial claims otherwise. I don't care how fancy the new gadget on late night TV appears to be. I don't care how much some famous celebrity was paid to tell you a new gimmick or "recently discovered secret" will get you fit in ten days. These are all unscientific claims and clever marketing ploys intended to sell products.

I only care to tell you the truth. This truth has worked for me and many, many others. Following the guidelines for diet and exercise described in this book, you should begin to FEEL positive effects after only a few weeks. You will begin to SEE significant physical improvements around the 12–16 week timeframe.

Consistency is Key for Older Individuals

It is time for another comparison of your body to an automobile. When we buy a new car, it continues to look good for the first few years regardless of how often we wash or wax it. The interior looks and smells like new for the first two or three years. But with the passage of time, the sun and elements combined with daily driving introduce wear and tear on the vehicle. By the time it reaches 8–10 years old, even the best kept car begins to shine a bit less, smell different, and has an interior that does not seem as luxurious.

Now, we all know plenty of older cars that look magnificent. The vehicles displayed at car shows prove that an automobile can still be in great shape 40 or 50 years later. BUT, this does not happen automatically. Those old cars need a lot of repair, washing, waxing, detailing, and TLC to be in such great shape at that age.

Hopefully by now you are encouraged by how much improvement you can make in your health and appearance in the second half of life. We said earlier that being over 40 was not over the hill as long as we lived a little smarter.

Consistency is one place where this smarter living idea comes into play. I am not going to sugar coat the truth here—you have to make the diet and exercise regimen described in this book a permanent part of your everyday lifestyle or you will not achieve the results you desire.

We can make amazing progress in our fitness as we age, but likewise, if we get apathetic or inconsistent it is easier to slip backwards. I know this firsthand. I follow the exact procedures described in this book in my own life.

Others who have used this information have told me it was the most straightforward advice they ever had, and it really worked for them. As I said earlier, this is one of the reasons I wrote this book—it works.

But I also know if I slack off or get sloppy in my eating habits, I can easily gain weight much faster than I did 30 years ago. If I go on a cruise with my wife and spend too much time at the buffet, I can easily gain 3–5 pounds in 7–14 days. It will take at least 2 weeks to remove that extra weight when I get home.

Think also of your personal automobile versus a car placed in a junkyard. This is a phenomenon that has always amazed me. You may have a car that sits outside year round in the rain, sun, and snow. Yet it still functions, holds up pretty well, and takes you anyplace you wish to go.

But look at a similar car parked in a junkyard. It is exposed to the same weather and elements, but after only a year, the car is rotting, faded, and appears to have been sitting in the field for 10–12 years.

With age, Father Time is constantly pushing us forward. Our combination of diet and exercise will not totally defeat these forces of nature or fully halt the passage of time. The best we can accomplish is to slow down the effects of biological aging as compared to the vast majority of sedentary or otherwise self-destructive people that surround us in modern society.

The popular phrase "use it or lose it" takes on added meaning for the over-40 person trying to stay in shape. We lose conditioning easier and faster in later years if we fall back on our bad habits. We can get in surprisingly good shape in our later years, but we have to be consistent.

✦ Important Principle ✦

Consistency is of Vital Importance for the older individual.

Diet and Exercise work wonders at slowing Father Time and allowing the body to maintain healthy function. But if we stray from our healthy regimen, the older body will lose conditioning much faster than a younger body. **Stay With It.**

It's impossible to stay consistent at something until you have actually started doing it in the first place.

With that thought in mind, let us end this chapter and get started with our first exercise routine.

Chapter Five

Getting Started

The 30–3 Routine

I have this theory that one day scientists will learn that the number 3 is somehow connected to the secrets of the universe.

Kepler's Three Laws of Planetary Motion
Third time is a charm
Celebrities die in threes
Three strikes and you're out
An atom has three constituents – protons, electrons, neutrons
Three Ring Circus
Three Blind Mice
Three is a Crowd
A Yard equals three feet
There are three notes in a simple musical chord
Three Little Pigs
The Three Wise Men
Newton's three Laws of Motion
Three branches of government
The three sources of calories are protein, carbohydrates, and fats

There are probably as least a hundred other examples that could be added to this list.

Is this coincidence, man's self-fulfilling prophecy, or some hidden code that explains the key to all existence?

Seriously, I don't know if there is really any special magic to the number three, or mankind has simply placed a special significance to it. Whatever the case, the number 3 and multiples of three will be a common theme in our exercise routines to follow.

The 30-3 Full Body & Cardio Routine

Some readers may already be exercising to some degree while others may not have been physically active in some time. In either case, when switching to a new form of physical activity it is wise to lay a foundation of conditioning before moving on to the more advanced regimens.

It is impossible to know the specific and unique physical and medical conditions of every person who may read these words. For that reason, you are urged to show this book to your doctor and discuss the exercises you plan to perform to ensure you have no special conditions that would make the suggested regimen inappropriate for you.

The 30-3 routine is a full body workout intended to serve as a general conditioning and foundation regimen. This routine includes the following features:

- Performed 3 days per week.
- Each major body part is trained with 3 working sets of a single exercise.
- 30 minutes of cardiovascular training.

This is an excellent routine in its own right for general conditioning. In fact, some people may be content with the benefits they see from this routine alone. For most people, this routine will be performed for a short period of time before moving to the full scale routine described in the next chapter.

How long should this 30-3 routine be used before moving on to our full scale 3 Day Per Week Split Routine? This answer will vary depending on your individual condition and doctor's advice, but as a general rule:

- If you have been physically active with a regular exercise routine until now and are simply trying something new, chances are you are in pretty good condition. You will only need to perform the 30-3 routine for 1–2 months before moving on to the Split Routine described in the next chapter.

- If you have been inactive and sedentary for some length of time and are only now embarking on a lifestyle change to improve your diet and exercise habits, you should use this 30-3 routine for at least 2–3 months before moving to the next level. Your doctor will most likely have his own recommendation regarding your progress.

Following are the details of the weight training regimen, descriptions of the exercises, and suggestions for the cardiovascular portion of your training.

At the end of the chapter, the entire regimen will be summarized in a quick reference summary page that you can copy and carry with you to the gym as a guide until you have your new routine memorized.

The 30-3 Weight Resistance Training Details

You will be performing one exercise for each major body part. You will begin by doing a warm up set of 15–20 repetitions with a light weight.

The purpose of this light set is to get the muscles, joints, and connective tissue warmed up and acclimated to the angle and range of motion before being subjected to a working load. Afterwards, you will perform 3 working sets of 12 reps, then 10 reps, then 8 reps.

You should increase the weight slightly every time you move to a set with lower repetitions. For example, this may be what the biceps portion of the regimen looks like:

Biceps Dumbbell Curl:

Warm-up Set	8 pounds	20 reps
Working Set 1	15 pounds	12 reps
Working Set 2	20 pounds	10 reps
Working Set 3	25 pounds	8 reps

You will then immediately move to the next body part.

Remember the rule for selecting the proper amount of weight is to select an amount that allows you to just barely complete the desired number of reps before reaching a point of failure.

In the example above, when performing Working Set 3 for 8 repetitions, you should just barely be able to complete the final repetition using proper form. The idea of trying to continue onward with 10–12, or more reps should seem very difficult or even almost impossible. If however you easily zip through all the working sets and have not needed to exert some concentrated effort to finish the last 1–2 reps in each set, then you are using too little weight.

You will be working the body in the following order:
• Warm-Up
• Chest
• Shoulders
• Triceps
• Back
• Biceps
• Quadriceps (front of leg)
• Hamstrings (back of leg)
• Calves
• Midsection

Following are the descriptions of the exercises for each body part itself. For most of the exercises in this book, I will attempt to include several alternatives of the same basic movement. These options are useful since different gyms may be equipped with different equipment.

Additionally, you may find a certain piece of equipment being used by another individual. Being familiar with your choices for alternative exercises that offer the same benefit can eliminate the frustration of waiting. Lastly, it is a good idea to introduce some variety into your exercise routine. Variety will allow the muscles to be exercised from slightly different angles while also helping prevent mental boredom.

WARM-UP

With age, our joints, spine, and connective tissue usually betray the wear and tear of decades long before the muscle tissue itself. For this reason, we want to perform a short warm up routine prior to any strength training exercises.

This series of warm up movements takes less than 5 minutes to perform, and is highly recommended before any strenuous physical exertion.

In fact, if I know I have a full day of yard work ahead of me, I will do this same quick loosening up routine before I grab the wheel barrows, rakes, and shovels.

Shoulder Rotations

Starting Position
Stand with your arms down by your side.

Movement
1. Slowly rotate your arm in a full forward circular motion.

2. As your hand lowers and begins to rotate behind your body, you will need to rotate the wrist. Be sure to rotate the arm through the shoulder's full range of natural motion.

4. Perform the desired number of repetitions. Repeat for the left arm.

5. Repeat the procedure for both arms by rotating the arms in the reverse direction.

Comments

Slow rotation is the important thing to remember with this warm up movement. The focus here is to ensure the shoulder joint and rotator cuffs are flexible and ready for subsequent exercises that require exertion. Do not spin the arms rapidly as you may have done when you were a young child pretending to be an airplane propeller.

(Photo 5.1) Shoulder rotations (sometimes called windmills) should be performed in a slow, full range of motion. No wild, fast swinging.

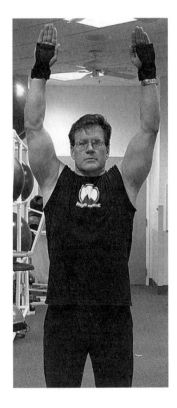

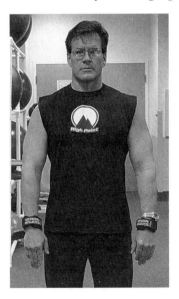

Some people prefer to rotate both arms at the same time. Either option is acceptable.

Arm & Elbow Stretches

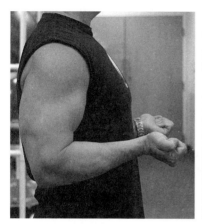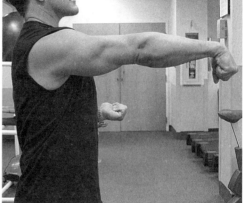

(Photo 5.2) The benefit of this warm up movement exists in the subtle details regarding elbow and wrist motion.

Starting Position
Stand with your arms and hands positioned as shown in the photo above. The position is similar to how your hands would be held if supporting a heavy tray close to the front of your body. You should have your wrists bent backwards as far as is comfortable such that you feel a mild stretch in the wrists and forearms.

Movement
1. Slowly extend your right arm forward as though you are throwing a punch in slow motion.

2. As your hand moves forward, rotate your wrist so that when you reach full extension, your fist is in a palm downward position.

3. Hold this extended position as you tilt your wrist forward and downward toward the floor. You should feel a nice stretch along the top of your forearm extending all the way back to your outer elbow region.

4. Reverse the motion, bringing your arm back to the starting position. You should also rotate your wrists so that by the time your arms are withdrawn, your hands are again in the starting position.

Comments

This is a stretching and warm up exercise that is a bit difficult to accurately describe in a book. Some people may emulate the general motion, but fail to feel the desired stretching in the wrists, elbows, and forearms. The key to getting benefit from this motion is to ensure that the wrists are flexed as far as possible until you can feel the gentle stretching extend all the way from the wrists to the elbows.

This motion is similar to a common therapy exercise for people suffering from elbow tendonitis. The benefit to us is that this motion prepares the elbows and wrists for weight-bearing exercises such as pushups, triceps dips, and other movements.

Wrist Rotations

Starting Position
Stand with your elbows bent at a 90 degree angle and your hands in front of your body.

Movement
1. This movement is very simple. Just rotate both wrists for 10–12 repetitions. Most people find it easier to rotate the wrists in opposite directions from each other, such that they are rotating like mirror images of each other.

2. Repeat in the opposite directions.

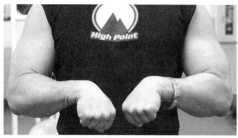
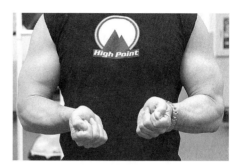

(Photo 5.3) Wrist Rotations.

Comments

This is a very simple motion, but it can be very beneficial to prevent injury. With age, some people complain that their wrists and ankles "get hung up" or otherwise click and pop when working under a load. This gentle warm up motion performed immediately before hard work tends to loosen the wrists and prevent them from experiencing this problem.

Lower Back Stretch

Starting Position

Stand in front of a chair or similar support. Hold the top of the chair for support. Step backwards approximately 3 feet until your arms are straight and you are bending forward slightly.

Movement

1. To stretch the right half of your lower back, drop your left knee slightly while also bending your left arm. This will allow your body to lean to the left and slightly forward (you might think of your head as pointing at the 10–11 o'clock position).

2. As your body leans to the left, your left leg will begin to support more of your bodyweight. You should feel a gentle stretch in the lower back of your right side. When you are in the proper stretched

position, your right foot should be slightly forward and resting on the heel. At this point, your right foot will be supporting very little of your bodyweight.

3. Focus on the gentle stretch in your lower back's right side.

4. Repeat this gentle stretching motion 2–3 times before mirror imaging the motion for your left side.

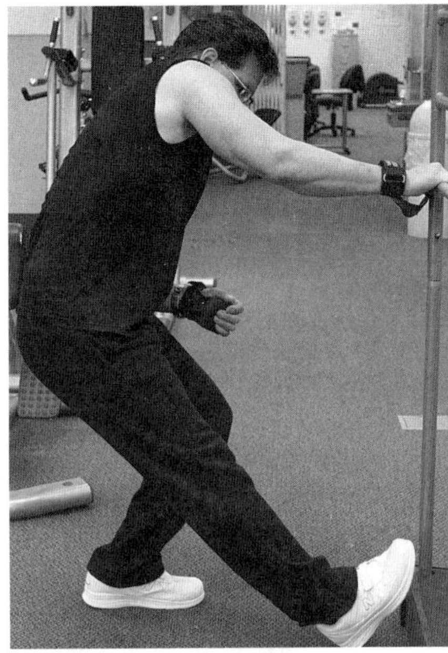

Comments

This is another stretching motion that is easier to demonstrate in a video or in person as compared to a book description.

(Photo 5.4)
Lower Back Stretch Movement

Even the picture above might make it a little difficult to understand the motion, but once you find the right position, you will know it.

Friends of mine with lower back problems or occasional sciatic twinges tell me this helps them loosen up their back before a day of hard work or other physical activity.

Leg and Knee Stretch

Starting Position

Stand in front of the same chair or support used in the previous movement. Hold the top of the chair (or support) with both hands for stability.

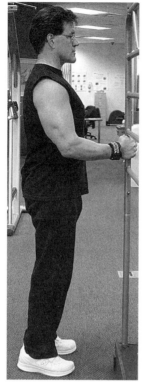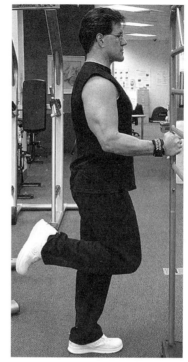

(Photo 5.5) Leg and Knee Stretch

Movement

1. Using the chair back to maintain your balance, slowly bend your right leg up behind you as far as possible. Imagine you are trying to touch your heel to your buttocks.

2. Slowly return your leg to the lower position.

3. In the lower position, tense your frontal thigh muscle while keeping your foot off the floor.

4. Repeat 6–10 repetitions. Do not allow your right foot to return to the floor until you are finished stretching this side.

5. Repeat for the left leg.

Comments

This simple motion limbers up the knees, hamstrings, and frontal thigh for later exercises.

Ankle Rotations

Starting Position

Stand in front of the same chair or support used in the previous two movements. Hold the top of the chair (or support) with both hands for stability.

Movement

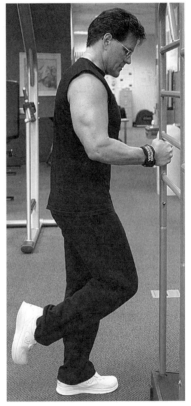

1. Lift your right foot slightly off the floor.

2. Rotate your ankle 10 times in a clockwise motion.

3. Repeat the rotation in a counter-clockwise direction.

4. Repeat for the left ankle.

Comments

A very simple warm up motion that helps prevent unexpected twisting or collapse of the ankle when walking, running, or doing exercises.

(Photo 5.6) Ankle Rotations

Calf and Achilles Tendon Stretch

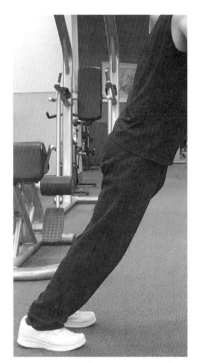 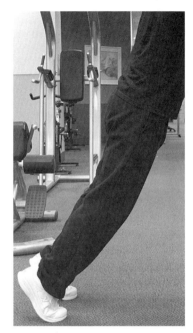

(Photo 5.7) Calf and Achilles Tendon Stretch

Starting Position

Stand with your feet approximately shoulder width apart. Place your hands on a wall for support. Step backwards approximately 3 feet from the wall so that you are leaning forward into the wall. Keep your feet flat on the floor. At this point you should feel a slight stretch to the back of your calves.

Movement

1. Slowly rise up on the balls of your feet while using the wall for support and balance.

2. Slowly lower your heels back to the floor allowing the Achilles tendon, gastrocnemius, and soleus muscles of the lower leg (calves) to stretch.

3. Repeat 10 repetitions or until you no longer feel any tightness in your lower legs.

Comments

With age, it is more important to keep the calves and Achilles tendon flexible to prevent tears or rupture. Let me relate a story that helps stress this point. I knew a man in his mid 40s who was in pretty good shape. He was visiting some friends who lived up North in the mountains. They had been riding through the woods on ATV vehicles for most of the day in 40 degree weather. Their exploration brought them to the foot of a mountain overlook.

The entire group jumped off their vehicles and began running up the steep slope of the mountainside in a quest to reach the spot that promised beautiful views of the valley below. Less than five strides after jumping off his ATV, this man felt he had been shot in the lower leg. His lower leg turned dark purple and swelled to almost double its normal size. He was unable to walk on the injured leg unless he slowly limped along on his tiptoes.

What was the diagnosis? He had torn a calf muscle. This pain continued for over a month. Why do I know this story so well? Time for a confession—I was that man!

This was one of the few major injuries I have experienced in my life. It resulted from being a bit reckless and forgetting my own fitness advice. Obviously, after spending a whole day sitting in a cool climate, I should have performed some simple stretching movements before jumping off a vehicle and running up the side of a steep mountain slope at full speed. Excitement had made me forget my own healthy habits that day.

What is the moral of this story? At 40 years old and older, we are not the same flexible creatures we were at age 12. Take 3–5 minutes to warm up and stretch your muscles and joints before taking on physical exertion. It is a small amount of time well spent.

If you are now warmed up, it is time to get started with the weight resistance portion of today's training.

CHEST

With age, our pectoral (chest) muscles tend to sag and weaken. This is largely due to gravity and the fact that many of us lead lives that do not require us to routinely perform many pressing motions.

The chest muscles are activated when we press outwards (similar to a push up or shoving somebody away from us). They are also utilized when we cross our arms in front of our body like a bear hug (this fact will be utilized later).

Our exercise for chest will be a form of incline press. The incline press will place more emphasis on the upper half of your chest and tend to give some lift to the chest region.

Later, when you progress to a split training routine, more exercises will be introduced to more fully work the chest from different angles. For now, our objective is to build a foundation by focusing on the region of the chest that is the least conditioned in most people.

Choose **one** of the exercises demonstrated below.

You will be performing 1 warm up set of 20 reps following by 3 working sets of 12-10-8 reps.

Several variations are provided to allow you flexibility based on the equipment available to you at your facility.

Incline Barbell Press

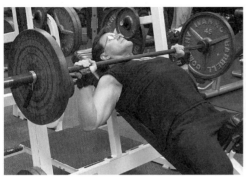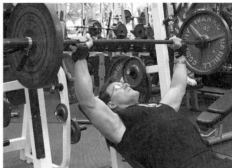

(Photo 5.8) Incline Barbell Press for Chest

Starting Position

Lay on a bench set to a 30–45 degree angle. Reach up and grab the bar approximately 3–5 inches wider than your shoulders. Keep your shoulders back with your chest forward.

Movement

1. Lower the weight in a slow, controlled motion so that the bar barely touches your upper chest 2–3 inches below your chin.

2. With slight accelerated force, push the barbell upwards until your elbows are almost straight. Do NOT lock out your elbows. Be sure your shoulders remain pulled back during the full motion.

Comments

In the lowered position, you forearms should be straight up and down in a perpendicular position under the bar. If you see that your wrists are not directly above your elbows, but are flared inwards or outwards, your beginning hand position was either too narrow or too wide.

A common mistake with chest pressing motions is the tendency to exaggerate the motion by pushing the shoulders forward and sinking in with the chest. Once the shoulders move in front of the chest, the frontal deltoid begins doing most of the work and the chest muscles are removed from the equation. Keep the shoulders pulled back and the chest out during the entire motion. You should feel the work being performed by your chest and not the front of your shoulders.

If your bench is adjustable, it is a good idea to vary the position of the backrest to work the chest at slightly different angles each day you train.

Incline Dumbbell Press

Starting Position
Sit on an incline bench that is set to a 30–45 degree angle. Allow the dumbbells to rest on your knees. Gently rock backward on the padded backrest of the bench while simultaneously bringing the weights up to shoulder level. As you bring the dumbbells off your knees and into their starting position, you should rotate the weights so that your hands are now palms forward in the starting position.

Movement
1. Keeping your shoulders pulled back and chest forward, press the weights upward. Stop just short of locking out your elbow joint.

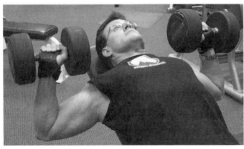

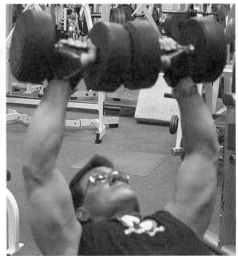

(Photo 5.9)
Incline Dumbbell Press for Chest

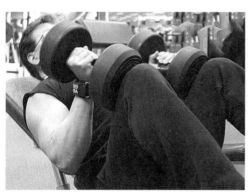
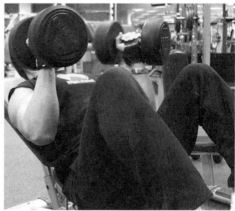

(Photo 5.10) Using legs to help get weights into the starting position.

2. Slowly lower the weights downward and slightly out to the sides as you return to the starting position.

Comments

If you find it difficult to get the dumbbells into their starting position, you can use your knees to help lift the weights up to your shoulders (Photo 5.10).

While the standard description for this exercise states that the hands should be in a palms forward direction, it is common to see some small variation in real life. This is especially true for those of us with slightly older bodies.

As we have already stressed, it is important to always perform our weight training exercises in a manner that follows a natural and full range of motion. For many people, trying to lift the dumbbells in a strict palms forward position may be slightly uncomfortable and could place extra stress on the joints. For many people (myself included), the motion feels more natural when the wrists are slightly turned at an 11 o'clock and 1 o'clock position (Photo 5.11).

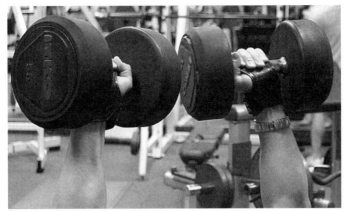

(Photo 5.11) Palms forward is an approximate description of hand position. Notice the more natural hand position exhibits a slight angle in some people.

Here is a quick and easy test you can do right now:
Quickly, without giving it much thought, close your right and left hands and extend your index finger and thumb as though you are making a gun. Now, stick both your arms out in front of you with the intention of holding these "gun hands" in a palms downward position.

Now look at your hands. Are your thumbs pointing perfectly parallel to the floor in the 3 and 9 o'clock positions? –OR–
Are your thumbs slightly higher than the pinky side of your hand, with the thumb pointing closer to the 1 and 11 o'clock positions?

This simple test demonstrates how a perfectly strict palms forward (or downward) position may or may not be 100% natural for you.

As soon as you have performed your warm up set and 3 working sets of the selected chest exercise, it is time to immediately move to shoulders.

SHOULDERS

Strong, wide shoulders have been a desired trait for men throughout all time. Women also now realize the advantages of having firm, fit shoulders, as they look nice in a sleeveless blouse. For both sexes, strong shoulders help with everyday activities like lifting objects and placing items on high shelves around the home.

Again, you will select **one** of the exercises demonstrated below.

As with most of our exercises, you will be performing 1 warm up set of 20 reps following by 3 working sets of 12-10-8 reps.

Variations are provided to allow you flexibility based on the equipment available to you at your facility.

Machine Shoulder Press

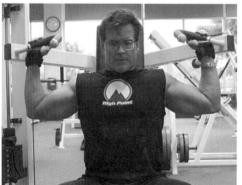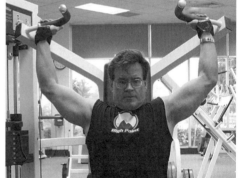

(Photo 5.12) Machine Press for Shoulders

Starting Position

Adjust seat so that the handles on either side of your head are approximately at ear level. The handles should also be near the middle of your head on either side. Keep feet firmly on the ground and your back erect against the seatback. Keep your elbows directly beneath the bar throughout your set.

Movement

1. Using your shoulder strength, press the handles upward until your elbows are just short of being locked out straight.

2. Slowly lower the bar back to the starting position with hands at approximately ear level.

Comments

You will notice we stressed a starting position that has your hands at approximately ear level. The reason for this is to always utilize lifting motions that allow the body to follow its natural range of motion.

You may see some people lowering the bar down below their chins when they perform this exercise. This is not a desirable practice. Such an extended range of motion takes the primary load off the deltoid muscles and can also introduce strain on the wrists and rotator cuff.

Time for another quick test. As you read these words, lift one of your arms up as though you are a waiter carrying a tray or are preparing to lift a log over your head. Where does your hand naturally fall? Chances are you now look similar to Photo 5.13.

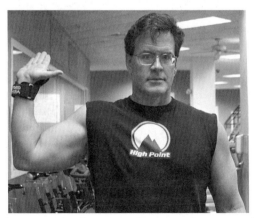

(Photo 5.13) The natural range of motion of the shoulder helps demonstrate our choice of starting position for the shoulder press exercise.

As was the case with chest presses, your forearms should be in a vertical position when performing this exercise. This means your elbows should be directly beneath your wrists as you lift the weights. Think of your forearms being like an old NASA rocket flying straight upwards through the ceiling. If you find your forearms are angled inwards or outwards when doing shoulder presses, you are using a hand grip that is either too narrow or too wide.

Dumbbell Shoulder Press

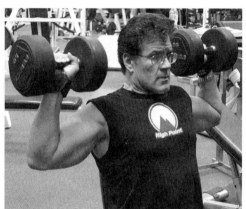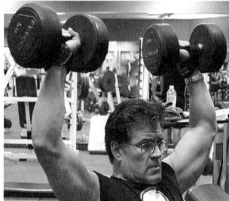

(Photo 5.14) Dumbbell Press for Shoulders

Starting Position
Grasp two dumbbells while sitting on a pressing chair that features a support for the lower back. Let the dumbbells rest on your knees as you sit down. Bring the dumbbells up to a starting position where each weight is held on either side of the head at approximately ear level. Your hands should be in a palms forward position.

Movement
1. Using your shoulder strength, press the dumbbells upward until your elbows are just short of being locked out straight.

2. Slowly lower the weights back to the starting position with hands at approximately ear level.

Comments

This exercise calls for a palms forward position. From our earlier explanation, it should be understood that this is intended to describe the basic hand position to be used. Anatomically each individual may exhibit a few degrees of rotation away from a strict palms forward position.

At the risk of sounding repetitive, you must always pay attention to your individual body's joint angles and range of motion. In real life, and especially after 40, 50, 60 or more years of wear and tear, it is natural for us to have a natural range of motion that varies slightly from a perfect textbook description.

You will notice in the accompanying photograph demonstrating this exercise (Photo 5.14), the hands are essentially in a palms forward position although a slight angle can be detected.

TRICEPS

When people think about arms, the first muscle that normally comes to mind is the bicep. In actuality, the triceps muscles on the back of the arm make up 2/3 of the upper arm's total size.

With age, the back of the arm often loses conditioning before the front biceps region. Some theorize that the reason for this is because most everyday activities don't work the back of the arm as much as the front. Regardless of the reason, many men and most women over the age of 50 complain about their triceps being loose and saggy.

Once again, you will be performing 1 warm up set of 20 reps following by 3 working sets of 12-10-8 reps. Two options are provided to allow you flexibility based on the equipment available to you at your facility.

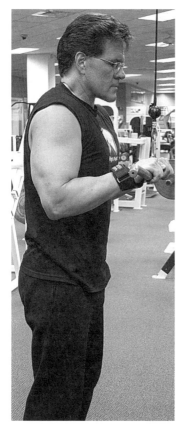 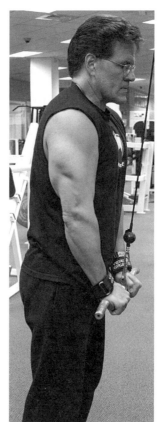

(Photo 5.15) Triceps Pulley Pushdowns

Triceps Pulley Pushdowns

Starting Position

Gyms normally have a wide variety of bars that are used with cable and pulley equipment. For triceps training, select the shorter handle that is angled downwards on the ends. This angled bar helps conform to the natural angle of the wrists when they are in the starting position for this exercise.

Adjust the height of the pulley such that when your elbows are at your sides, and you are holding the bar with an overhand grip, the bar is in

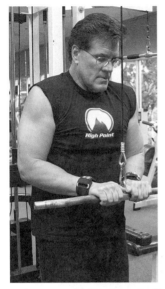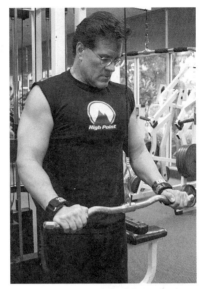

(Photo 5.16) Triceps Pulley Pushdowns varying hand position for changing target more to the inner or outer triceps.

the region of your upper chest.Using this overhand grip, your thumb will also be above the bar.

Movement

1. With your elbows kept in position on the sides of your body, press downward until your arms are just shy of being fully extended. By now you have probably noticed a common theme with our exercises. We never want to extend any joints into a fully-locked position. A fully-locked joint position takes workload off the muscles and places almost all the stress on the joints. This is something we wish to avoid when joint health preservation is of such vital importance.

2. Slowly return the bar to the starting position while insuring the elbows remain in position close to the sides of the body. You should feel the back of your arms doing 95% of the work.

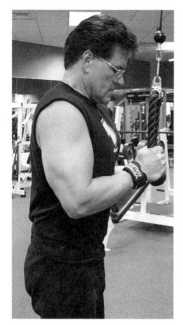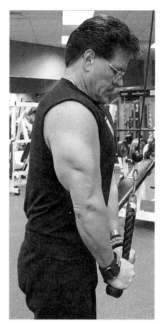

(Photo 5.17) Triceps Pulley Pushdowns using Rope Attachment for Variation

Comments

The back of the arm is called the triceps because it is actually composed of three muscles. The normal hand position with your elbows at the side and hands directed straight out in front of you is best for letting all three muscles of the triceps share in the work.

For variety, you can move your hands closer or farther out to help target the outer or inner portions of the triceps as you prefer (Photo 5.16). More variety can be introduced with this movement by using a rope attachment that allows the hands to maintain a "palms facing each other" orientation (Photo 5.17).

Each small variation in hand position should allow you to feel the work being performed in different areas of the rear arm. Try using some hand position variety each day you visit the gym to ensure all portions of your triceps get a good workout.

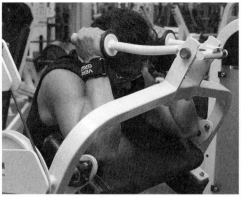
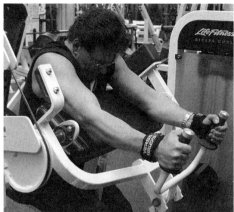

(Photo 5.18) Triceps Extension Machine

Triceps Extension Machine

Starting Position
Adjust the height of the seat so that your upper arms rest on the support pad. Sit down. If the height is properly adjusted, your elbows should be straight in front of you, with your upper arms approximately parallel to the ground. Grab the two handles and bend your arms fully while being sure your upper arms maintain contact with the support pad at all times. Most machines have a pivot point identified on the apparatus. The objective is to line up your movable joint with the pivot point. In this case, your elbow should be in line with the identified pivot point.

Movement
1. Using only triceps strength, slowly straighten your arms. Stop when your arms are just shy of being fully straight. As we have stressed so many times before, do not lock out your elbow joint.

Comments
Resist the natural urge to lift your upper arms off the support pad. If you allow your arms to lift off the pad to gain leverage, you will lose

much of the focused benefit of this exercise. You should really be able to feel the back of your arms working with this movement.

BACK

Keeping the upper back muscles strong will help you maintain proper posture, hold the body upright, and prevent the common tendency for older people to exhibit a hunched or stooped look. A health upper back will also minimize problems with spinal discomfort in the thoracic and cervical regions.

Again, you will select **one** of the exercises demonstrated below.

You will be performing 1 warm up set of 20 reps following by 3 working sets of 12-10-8 reps.

Variations are provided to allow you flexibility based on the equipment available to you at your facility.

Seated Pulley Rows

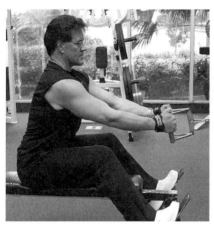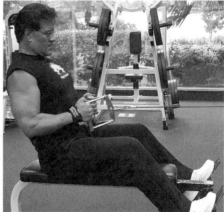

(Photo 5.19) Seated Pulley Rows.

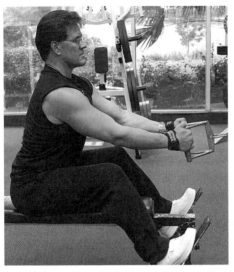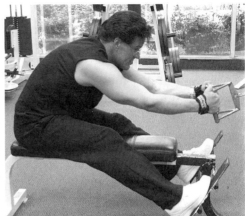

(Photo 5.20) A Comparison of Proper versus Improper lower back position when performing Seated Pulley Rows. Any forward body motion should come from rotation at the hip, not bending at the waist.

Starting Position

Most gyms will offer a variety of different handles for use with the seated pulley machine. These will range from a narrow V-shaped handle to a longer straight bar that feels more like rowing a boat oar. At this stage, select the V-shaped attachment, since it allows your hands to hold the handle in the more comfortable "palms facing each other" orientation.

Grab the bar and sit up straight with your shoulders pulled back. Place your knees on the platform with your knees slightly bent to offer stability. Keep your back arched in its anatomically preferred S position. Do NOT bend forward or allow your back to bow when lifting the weights (see Photo 5.20).

Movement

1. Without letting your shoulders shift forward, pull back on the cable attachment in a motion similar to rowing a boat. Your hands should touch your body near the bottom of your rib cage.

2. Slowly return the weight to the starting position. Be careful not to lean forward at the waist or allow your back to bow.

3. Repeat this rowing motion for the desired number of repetitions.

Comments

The hardest thing for people to learn with rowing and most back exercises is to let the back do the pulling, not the arms. You should think of your arms and hands as being nothing more than ropes and hooks that are holding the weights, while your back does the actual pulling.

Focus on feeling the back doing the work and not your upper arms. Once you find the right feel, you will better understand the point being made here.

Most people have a normal tendency to try to pull the weight back using their upper arms and forearms instead of their back. This tendency is most likely due to the average person not being involved in daily activities that use a rowing motion extensively.

Any forward bending motion should come from rotation at the hips and not bending at the waist.

Seated Machine Rows

Starting Position

You will find a variety of machines in most gyms that offer some variation of the seated row. Depending upon their design and angle, each may target one area of the back more than another. For our purposes with the 30-3 Routine, any of the machines that simulate the basic rowing motion will prove both acceptable and productive.

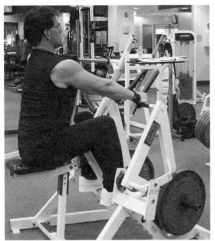
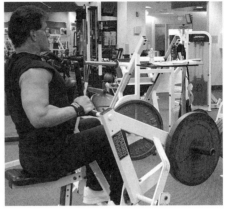

(Photo 5.21) The seated machine row is a variation of the seated pulley row described above.

The basic instruction of keeping your shoulders back, chest out, and back in a properly postured S-shaped arch holds true on the machines just as on the pulleys.

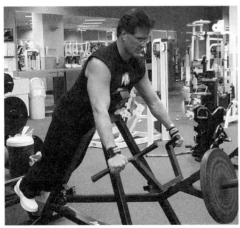
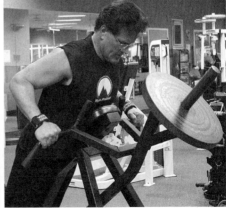

(Photo 5.22) Most gyms offer a variety of machines that offer a basic rowing motion.

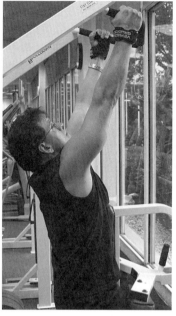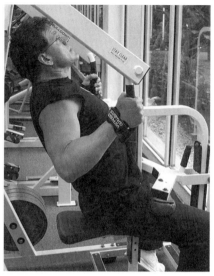

(Photo 5.23) While each rowing machine works the entire back, there are slight differences in the area targeted by each movement. Try a different rowing exercise each time you visit the gym for variety.

Movement

1. Without letting your shoulders shift forward, pull back on the machines handles in a motion similar to rowing a boat. Your hands should come close to touching your body near the top of the range of motion.

2. Slowly return the weight to the starting position. Be careful not to allow your back to bow.

3. Repeat this rowing motion for the desired number of repetitions.

Comments

If your gym offers seated pulley machines and also a wide variety of machines that provide a similar rowing motion, I suggest you mix it up each time you visit the gym. One visit, use the seated pulley. During the next visit, use one of the other machines.

Some machines will use a selectorized weight stack that allows you to easily select the desired weight with a pin. Other machines may require you to actually place plates of weight on either side. I have included a few examples of the types of machines you may have in your gym location (Photos 5.21–5.23).

Lat Cable Pulldowns

Starting Position
A wide variety of handle attachments can be used on the lat cable pulldown machine. For our purposes, we will be using a long 4' bar with slightly bent ends that will be a bit wider than your shoulders (see Photo 5.24).

Take an overhand grip on the bar 4–8 inches wider than your shoulders on each side. Straighten your arms just shy of being locked. (Remember we NEVER want to lock our joints when performing any weight-bearing exercise). Secure your knees under the restraint bar. This will prevent you from being lifted off your seat as you pull down on the weights.

The basic instruction of keeping your shoulders back, chest out, and back in a properly postured S-shaped arch holds true on the pulldown machine just as it did on the various rowing motions.

Movement
1. Lean slightly backwards, maintaining the healthy arch in your back.

2. Without letting your shoulders shift forward, pull back on the bar in a motion similar to doing a chin up, like you did in physical education class as a kid.

3. You should pull the bar down to a point somewhere between your chin and upper chest. The exact point where you stop pulling will

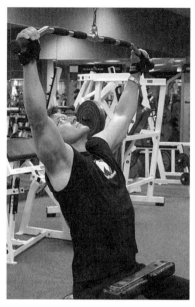
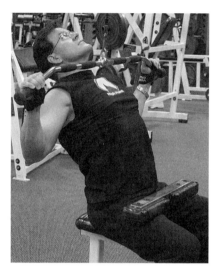

(Photo 5.24) Lat Cable pulldowns.

vary between individuals based on anatomical variation and range of motion capability.

4. Slowly return the weight to the starting position. Maintain the arched seated position with your upper body leaning slightly backwards. Be careful not to allow your back to bow or bend forward at the waist.

5. Repeat this pulldown motion for the desired number of repetitions.

Comments

At first glance it is clear to see that this exercise is quite different from the rowing motions we demonstrated earlier. The truth is, the back is a large and complex muscle group. No single exercise alone can fully exercise our backs from every angle and give us the full conditioning we desire.

You will most likely feel this pulldown exercise targeting the latissimus muscles of the back more than the various rowing motions. The latissimus muscles (lats) are the broad muscles of the upper back just posterior to the arm. In men, they are the muscles that offer the classic V shape to the torso. Firm lats on women help improve the appearance in swimsuits, formal gowns, and lacey tops.

When you advance to the full scale 3 Day Per Week Split Routine you will see that each back workout will use a combination of exercises to work the back from different angles. For now it should be kept in mind the 30-3 Routine is intended to be a foundation regimen to get the body generally conditioned.

Only one of the back exercises shown above should be selected each time you visit the gym. Ideally, you would like to mix it up and select something different each day you work out.

For example, suppose you are going to the gym on Tuesday, Thursday and Saturday each week following the 30-3 Routine being described in this chapter. On Tuesday, you may choose to do the Seated Pulley Rows. On Thursday, it would be smart to perform the Lat Cable Pulldowns to exercise the back from a different angle. On Saturday, you might use one of the rowing machines.

With the back exercise completed, it is time to move on to the biceps.

BICEPS

Ask anybody to "show me your muscles," and they will undoubtedly stick out their arm in the classic muscle man pose and flex their biceps muscle. The biceps is the muscle group on the front of the arm which is responsible for bending the arm and rotating the wrist.

When it comes to motivating people to exercise, most men are more than eager to work the biceps. Women often exhibit a preference for training their legs, but in recent years even the fairer sex has learned to appreciate the look and feel of a firmer and stronger upper arm.

Again, you will select **one** of the exercises demonstrated below.

You will be performing 1 warm up set of 20 reps following by 3 working sets of 12-10-8 reps.

Variations are provided to allow you flexibility based on the equipment available to you at your facility.

Biceps Barbell Curl

Starting Position
Place an appropriate amount of weight on a standard barbell. Be sure to use the locking collars provided by the gym as these will prevent the weights from sliding off the ends of the bar.

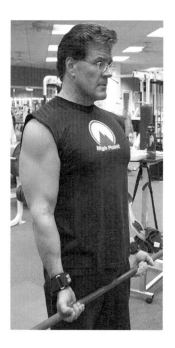
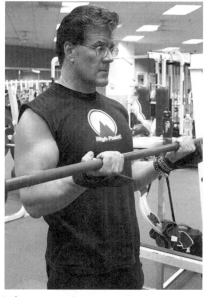

(Photo 5.25) Proper Biceps Barbell Curl Technique.

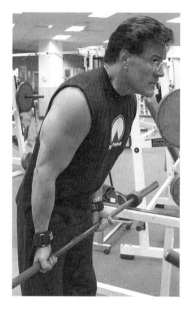 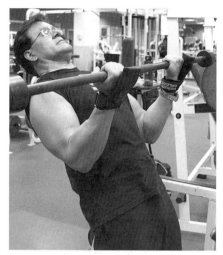

(Photo 5.26) Improper Rocking and Swaying of the Upper Body Is Often Caused By Using Too Much Weight.

With your feet in a comfortable and stable shoulder-width stance, grab the bar at a distance equal to where your arms naturally fall when they are dropped to your sides. You will more than likely find this distance to be approximately the same as shoulder width (see Photo 5.25). Your hands should be in a palms upward position as you grab the barbell.

Movement

1. Without swaying or leaning your torso in any way, use only your bicep strength to curl the barbell upwards. The barbell should be lifted to the highest point you can raise the bar without allowing your elbows to leave the side of your body.

2. Slowly return the bar to the lowered position with your elbows just shy of being fully extended. Do not fully relax or let the weight hang from your fully extended arms.

3. Repeat this motion for the desired number of repetitions.

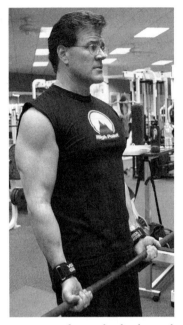
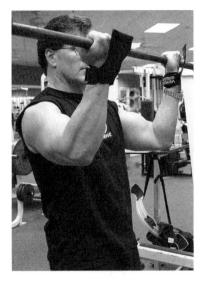

(Photo 5.27) Improper Biceps Curl. Note the elbows have been allowed to move away from the body and into a forward position. This mistake takes the focus off the biceps and allows the frontal shoulders to assume all the workload.

Once again, it is important to remember we never want to fully lock out any joints or take the load off the muscles when performing weight training exercises. I know this tip may seem repetitive by now, but it is very important to remember in order to successfully strengthen muscles but protect joints from injury.

Comments

The barbell curl is one of the most basic and effective ways to train the biceps muscle. Despite its apparently simple nature, there are three common mistakes you will see people make almost anytime you visit a gym.

First, people will use too heavy of a weight. When the weight is too heavy, they often develop a bad habit of swinging the weight and rock-

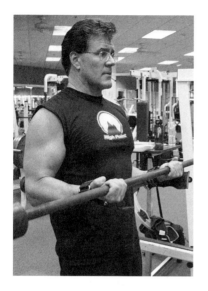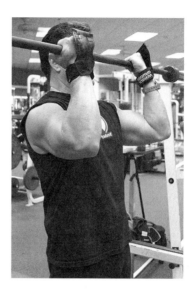

(Photo 5.28) Another example of an improper biceps curl. Note the elbows are never straightening out. There is no biceps action being performed here. The locked arms are simply being rotated and raised by the shoulders. This mistake in not only useless for the biceps muscle, but also increases the possibility of shoulder injuries.

ing their upper body to gain leverage and momentum against the load. This sloppy technique will take the focus and intensity off the biceps. Yes, a person can lift more weight when they start rocking and swaying their upper body, but that is only because the back, shoulders, legs, and trapezius muscles begin contributing to the effort (Photo 5.26).

Secondly, as the weight is curled upwards, people will move their arms forward such that the elbows leave the sides of the body. Once the elbows leave your side and extend in front of you, stress is taken off the biceps and the frontal deltoid (shoulder) muscle begins to do most of the work. People using this wrong technique will often bring the bar up close to their chins (Photo 5.27). If you use proper technique with your elbows locked to your sides, you will find that the hand can not reach much higher than chest level.

Lastly, another common problem often seen when people perform the curl is they do not straighten the arm at the elbow. Instead of using the bicep to raise and lower the forearm, they keep the arm locked in 90 degree angle and simply rotate the whole arm at the shoulder. This action does virtually NOTHING for the biceps muscle since there is no actual movement or action being performed with this flawed technique that even remotely reflects the natural action and functions of the biceps (Photo 5.28).

Earlier we spoke about hand angles when training the shoulders. The same advice is useful to remember when performing the barbell curl. Some individuals find a strict palms upward position to be uncomfortable. Some people may experience discomfort near their elbows. It is totally permissible to use a slightly natural rotation in the wrist when grabbing the bar if it is more comfortable.

For those with a history of forearm pain or tendonitis in the lateral or medial epicondyle (outer or inner elbow), using a slightly relaxed angle in the wrist as opposed to a tight and straight forearm grip is also a useful technique to use when exercising arms. This tip can help diminish the discomfort of tennis or golfer's elbow when exercising the arms (see Photo 5.29).

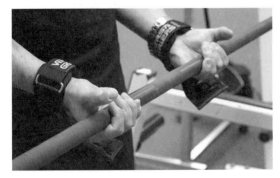

(Photo 5.29) Incorporating a slightly relaxed grip when exercising arms can be helpful to diminish discomfort for those suffering from tennis or golfer's elbow.

Cambered Bar Curls

Starting Position

Place an appropriate amount of weight on a cambered curl bar. Be sure to use the locking collars provided by the gym as these will prevent the weights from sliding off the ends of the bar.

With your feet in a comfortable and stable shoulder width stance, grab the bar at the spot where the handles curve and conform to a natural hand position.

You will find one such spot on the bar is close to shoulder width. A second spot to grab the bar will allow for a narrower grip. For our purposes, select the distance most close to matching your shoulder width (see Photo 5.30). Your hands should be in a palms upward position as you grab the barbell, although they will actually be rotated at a 20–30 degree angle.

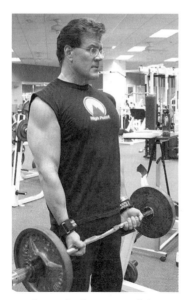
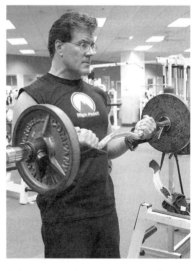

(Photo 5.30) Performing biceps curls with this curved bar can eliminate wrist discomfort for those who find the straight bar uncomfortable.

Movement

1. Without swaying or leaning your torso in any way, use only your bicep strength to curl the barbell upwards. The barbell should be lifted to the highest point you can raise the bar without letting your elbows leave the side of your body.

2. Slowly return the bar to the lowered position with your elbows just shy of being fully extended. Do not fully relax or let the weight hang from your fully extended arms.

3. Repeat this motion for the desired number of repetitions.

Once again it is important to remember we never want to fully lock out any joints or take the load off the muscles when performing weight training exercises. I know this tip may seem highly repetitive by now, but it is very important to remember if we wish to successfully strengthen muscles but protect joints from injury.

Comments

The biceps curl using the cambered bar is really just a modification of our standard straight barbell curl. It is potentially helpful enough for some people that it deserves its own unique description.

As explained earlier, the biceps muscle is responsible for raising the forearm and rotating the wrist. In fact, even if you do not flex your biceps, you can feel it contract into a small baseball shape simply by rotating your wrist.

In the comments regarding the standard barbell curl, we explained that some people with elbow or forearm pain may experience discomfort when using the straight barbell in a strict palms upward position. The tip was introduced to slightly rotate and relax the wrist to help alleviate this discomfort.

The cambered curl bar simply takes this remedy to the next step. Performing curls with the curved bar and rotated wrists will not work the bicep as directly as the straight bar. Despite being slightly less effective, this compromise may be necessary for those with elbow joint and forearm pain.

Dumbbell Curls

Starting Position
Grab two appropriately weighted dumbbells and stand with your feet positioned at a natural standing width.

Stand erect with your arms hanging down and holding a dumbbell at each side. Hold the dumbbells in a palms upward position. Press your upper arms against the sides of your body and keep them in this position throughout the full motion.

Movement
1. Without swaying your upper body, use only your biceps strength to curl your right arm upwards in an arc. Lift the weight as high as possible without removing your elbow from its position on the side of your torso.

2. As you lower the right dumbbell to its starting position, simultaneously begin lifting the left dumbbell to the raised position.

3. Continue performing this seesaw motion until you have performed the desired number of repetitions for each arm.

Comments
It is often helpful to hold the dumbbell closer to the end of the bar near your body in order to clear your hips while performing this exercise.

As with the barbell exercises, it is important to imagine a rod going through your body and holding the elbows in position on either side of your body. There is a natural tendency to try to lift the weights too high (near the chin). This habit causes the elbows to move forward. As ex-

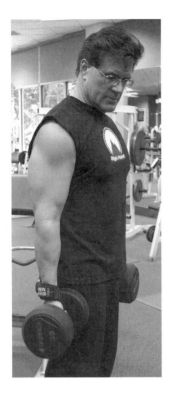
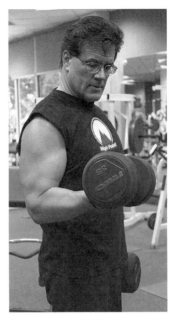

(Photo 5.31) Dumbbell Curls

plained earlier, once the elbows move forward in front of the body, focus is shifted from the biceps to the frontal deltoids.

Dumbbell curls lend themselves to a wide range of variations. They can be performed in either a standing or sitting position. You can also rotate the wrist midway through the motion to increase intensity on the flexed biceps muscle. Rotating the wrist while lifting offers the added benefit of exercising the biceps through both of its normal functions. The biceps will be worked through both motions of hand pronation-supination and flexing the arm.

With each arm able to move independently, you can also experiment with minor differences in how far outwards you hold the weight as you perform the curling motion. These variations will be explored in more depth when we advance to the 3 Day per Week Split Routine. For the first few months of your conditioning, alternating between the standard barbell and dumbbell curls described above will give you all the biceps stimulation you need to develop new strength and firmness.

That takes care of biceps. Now it is time to move onward to exercising the legs.

QUADRICEPS (front of leg)

As we get older, maintaining mobility and independence becomes very important to us. There is a big difference in the quality of life between those who are able to energetically move around in the world and those who find it difficult to stand or walk for any length of time.

Recent studies reveal that 33% of people over the age of 45 report having some type of knee pain. This statistic only increases with age as the effects of osteoarthritis, bursitis, and tendonitis take a greater hold on aging joints. These ailments tend to be more common in people who are overweight and/or have poor leg muscle development. Exercise also helps alleviate some of the problems experienced with knee pain by maintaining better flexibility in the joints.

When it comes to exercising the quadriceps muscles of the leg, we make a small change to our normal Sets and Repetition profile. Because the knees are such an important joint that also cause problems for many people over the age of 40 , we incorporate an extra exercise intended to warm up the knees before beginning the actual working motions.

Before choosing a primary lifting exercise, you will be doing 3 sets of an exercise called the Leg Extension. The Leg Extension is commonly used in rehabilitation programs for individuals who have experienced injury or surgery to their knees.

After performing 3 sets of lightweight leg extension warm ups, everything else will be the same as you have done with the other body parts.

You will select **one** of the exercises demonstrated below.

You will be performing 1 warm up set of 20 reps for the selected exercise, following by 3 working sets of 12-10-8 reps.

Variations are provided to allow you flexibility based on the equipment available to you at your facility.

Leg Extension Warm Up Exercise

Starting Position
Although there is a wide variety of different makes and models of leg extension machines available in gyms, they all allow for the same basic movement.

Sit in the machine with your back resting firmly against the backrest. Your knees should extend out over the edge of the seated area so that they can hang and move freely while the majority of your leg is supported by the seat. Most machines will feature a label that identifies the pivot point of motion for the machine. Your knee joint should be aligned with this pivot point.

Slip your ankles under the padded bar or roller pads. With your ankles flexed to form a 90 degree angle, the pad should rest comfortably in the angle of your flexed ankle. The pad should NOT be resting too high on the shins.

Select a relatively light weight that will allow you to perform 15–20 repetitions. Slide the selector pin into the weight stack.

While maintaining this sitting position, grab the handles on either side of the machine to stabilize the upper body.

Movement
1. Using the strength of your quadriceps muscle, straighten your legs in a steady motion such that they travel outward and upward. Stop the

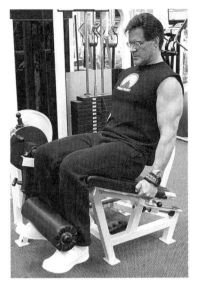

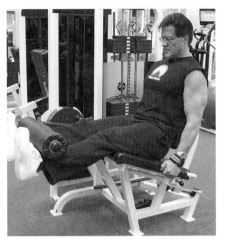

(Photo 5.32) Regardless of the quadriceps leg exercise you choose to perform, leg extensions should always be performed first as a warm up exercise for the knees.

upward motion when your legs are almost straight. Do not lock out your knee joints.

2. After maintaining this almost straightened leg position for a brief moment, slowly return the feet back downward to the starting position.

Comments

For our purposes, the leg extension should only be used as a warm up exercise to loosen up the knee and frontal leg muscles. Do NOT use an excessively heavy weight when performing this motion.

As mentioned in the introduction to this section, the leg extension exercise is a great movement that is often used as a rehabilitation movement following knee surgery or serious injury. Despite this fact, the knee does not normally get subjected to heavy forces when moving through this range of motion in everyday life. The natural work expected of the leg and knee joint is to allow us to stand up, walk, jump, run, and even kick.

The motion of kicking a soccer ball may be the closest "natural" activity we perform that is imitated by the leg extension exercise. Even in this example, kicking a one pound soccer ball from a running position is not exactly the same as sitting on a bench and lifting a heavy weight upwards by straightening the knee joint.

While visiting the gym, you may see some bodybuilders or other athletes use heavier weights when performing this exercise. For our goals, I will again stress that you should only use the leg extension as a warm up exercise to prepare your quadriceps and knees for harder work. Do not try to use heavy weights and low repetitions when performing this exercise.

Now that you have warmed up your knees with the leg extension, it is time to choose **one** of the following exercises to work the legs.

Angled Leg Press

Starting Position
Place an appropriate amount of weight on the leg press apparatus. Be sure to distribute the weight equally on both sides of the machine. Sit in the machine with your back resting firmly against the padded back support.

Place your feet on the platform approximately shoulder width apart. Orient your toes in a slightly outwards position. Straighten your legs and release the safety stops on either side of the machine.

Movement
1. Slowly lower the sliding platform by bending your knees. As your knees bend, be sure they remain oriented such that they point in the same direction as your toes. Lower the platform as low as possible while ensuring that your butt does not lift off the seat. For most

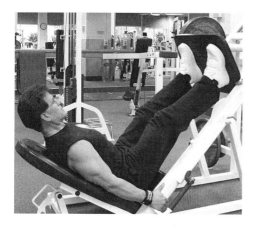

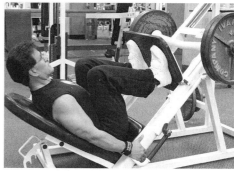

(Photo 5.33) Proper Technique Demonstration of the Angled Leg Press

people, this lowered position will produce an approximate 90–110 degree angle in the knee joint.

2. As soon as you have reached the lowered position, firmly press upward with your legs until your legs are almost straight. Do NOT lock the knees in the top position.

Comments

When lowering the weighted platform, it is important to get a full range of motion. It is very common to see people use far too much weight on

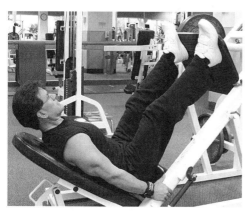

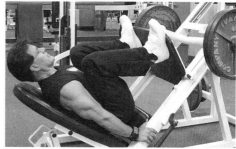

(Photo 5.34) Improper Angled Leg Press technique. Notice the buttocks are being raised off the seated support. This problem occurs when the weight is lowered too far, OR, the feet are placed too high on the platform.

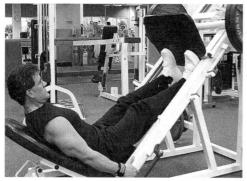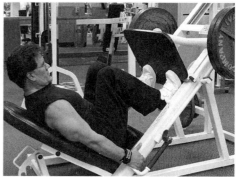

(Photo 5.35) Improper Angled Leg Press technique. Notice how the knees are extending outwards far past the toes. This mistake can add unwanted pressure to the knee joint. This problem occurs when the feet are placed too low on the platform.

the leg press, but only move their legs a few inches. This limited range of motion introduces almost no bend in the knee, fails to work the quadriceps, and also exposes the knee joint to potential injury.

The leg press also benefits your gluteal and hamstring muscles in addition to the front quadriceps.

The leg press is a classic example of an exercise where our mantra of *full and natural range of motion* is of critical import.

If you find your butt lifting off the seat in the lowered position, this is a sign that you are lowering the weight too far, OR, your feet are planted too high on the platform.

It is natural and acceptable for the knees to extend past the toes slightly when performing squatting motions, but when performing exercises under a load, we want to avoid exaggerating this position. If the knee extends far beyond the toes in a weight-loaded situation, it can increase sheer force in the knee joint.

The proper position of your feet on the platform will be somewhere near the middle section. This position will allow your knee to bend naturally and also allow your knees to extend only slightly beyond your toes when in the lowered position.

Seated Leg Press

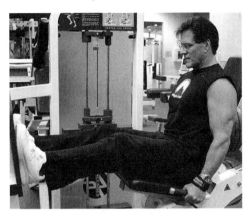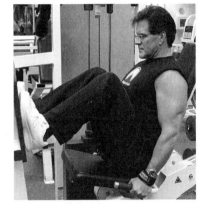

(Photo 5.36) Proper Technique Demonstration of the Seated Leg Press.

Starting Position

Sit in the machine with your back resting firmly against the padded back support. Place your feet on the platform approximately shoulder width apart. Orient your toes in a slightly outwards position. Choose an appropriate amount of weight using the pin selector.

Set the adjustment lever such that your legs can travel a full range of motion from fully bent to just shy of totally straight.

Grasp the handles on either side of the seat for stability while keeping your back firmly pressed against the padded support.

Movement

1. Slowly bend your legs as fully as is comfortable while being sure your buttocks and back do not leave the seat and rear support. For most people this will translate to a bend in the knee of 90–110 degrees. Your knees should travel slightly out to your sides as opposed to

pressing against your stomach. This path of motion along the sides of your body will allow for a larger range of leg movement.

2. Without jerking or bouncing the weight in any way, reverse the direction of movement by pressing forward with your frontal leg muscles. As you press the platform forward, you should stop when your legs are almost fully straight, but the knee joint is NOT locked.

Comments
The seated leg press is essentially a variation of the angled leg press. The seated leg press offers the convenience of not needing to load free weight plates. The upright seated position is also more comfortable for some people.

The seated leg press, however, does not offer the same extra benefit to the gluteal and hamstring muscles as does the angled leg press. As we have mentioned many times already, your best results will come from incorporating variety in your routine. If you have no personal injuries or handicaps that prevent you from performing the different types of leg presses, you should make a point of alternating between the different machines every so often.

Several manufactures produce their own version of the seated leg press machine. You may in fact find more than one type in your own gym. On some models the seat moves while the foot platform remains stationary. Other models allow the foot platform to move while the seat remained fixed. Regardless of these variations, they all allow for the same basic movement.

At this point, you have just finished 3 warm up sets of leg extensions followed by a warm up set of leg presses and 3 working sets of leg presses.

It is time to move to the back of the leg and exercise the hamstrings.

HAMSTRINGS (back of leg)

Unlike the quadriceps which get lots of attention, the hamstrings are often not given much thought by most people until they get injured or strained. The hamstrings run along the backside of your leg between your knee and buttocks. Along with your quadriceps, they play a key role in supporting your knee joint. Healthy, flexible hamstrings are important for bending, walking, climbing, and performing common everyday activities such as dressing.

Failure to exercise the hamstrings while only strengthening the quadriceps can create a muscle imbalance in the leg that can contribute to knee instability and joint pain. The 30-3 Routine you are doing now as well as the 3 Day per Week Split Routine you will begin performing in a few months is designed to condition all your major muscle groups to an equal degree.

Again, you will select **one** of the exercises demonstrated below.

You will be performing 1 warm up set of 20 reps following by 3 working sets of 12-10-8 reps.

Variations are provided to allow you flexibility based on the equipment available to you at your facility.

Lying Leg Curl

Starting Position
Lie facedown on the padded surface of the machine. Your knees should be just off the edge of the bench such that no pressure is applied on the knee cap when the movement is performed.

Place your heels under the roller pads. When your feet are pointed directly forward, the roller pad should rest on your ankles near the heel. If

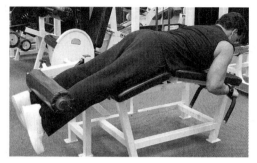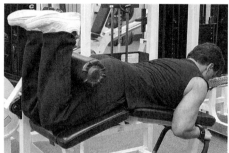

(Photo 5.37) Lying Leg Curls

the bar is hitting too high on the lower leg near the calf region, use the adjustment screw to set the machine to proper length.

Grasp the handles near the head end of the padded surface to stabilize your torso.

Movement

1. While making sure your hips do not rise off the surface of the machine, use your hamstring (leg bicep) muscle to move your feet upward in an arc motion until you feel the back of your legs fully contracted. For many people this means the roller pad will lightly bump into the buttocks region in the topmost position.

2. Slowly return the feet to the starting position along this same semi-circular arc movement.

3. Perform this full range of movement for the desired number of repetitions.

Comments

A common mistake seen with people performing the lying leg curl is that they raise their hips off the bench. "Cheating" in this way takes the focus off the hamstring and allows other muscles to contribute to the lifting effort. Those individuals who lay flat on the bench are most often guilty of this error.

One effective way to prevent the hips from lifting off the bench is to elevate the chest slightly when performing this movement. This is most easily accomplished by resting your upper body on the forearms or using the machine's support handles in a manner similar to a racing bicycle. This technique is used in the demonstration photograph for this exercise (see Photo 5.37).

Seated Leg Curls

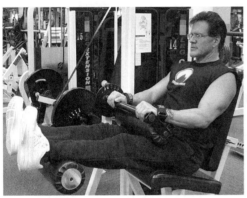

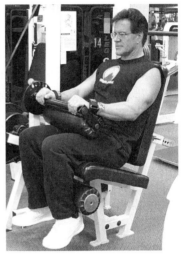

(Photo 5.38) Seated Leg Curls

Starting Position

The roller pads on seated leg curl machines can be adjusted to match the length of your legs. When you sit in the machine with your toes pointed straight upwards toward the ceiling, the roller pads should rest on the back of your ankle near the heel.

When properly adjusted for your size, lower the restraint bar so that it rests on your thighs. The fit should be snug enough to prevent your legs from being lifted off the seat when performing the motion.

Movement

1. Using only the strength of your hamstrings muscles and keeping your ankles flexed in a toes forward position, contract the leg biceps

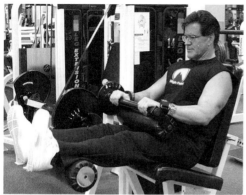
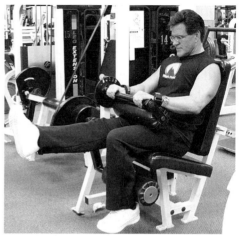

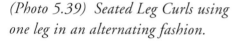
(Photo 5.39) Seated Leg Curls using one leg in an alternating fashion.

to bring the heels down in an arc motion. When fully contracted, you will feel the tension in the back of your legs. Your feet will now be beneath you on the seat.

2. Slowly allow the roller pad to return upwards to the starting position. Stop the motion just shy of being fully straight so that the knee joint is not allowed to fully lock, and tension is maintained on the hamstrings.

3. Repeat this motion for the desired number of repetitions.

Comments

Some people find it beneficial to perform this exercise using only one leg at a time. When doing the seated leg curl in this manner, you hold one leg up in the air while the other leg exerts the effort. When you return to the top starting position, you alternate legs and continue performing this motion in a seesaw fashion. The full exercise assumes a "walking through the air" appearance when performed in this manner (see Photo 5.39).

Obviously, less weight will be used when only one leg is worked at a time. Additionally, extra caution should be used to hold the upper body stable and not allow the torso to twist in such a way that injury or discomfort results.

With the hamstrings now exercised, it is time to do some work for the calf muscles of the lower leg.

CALVES

What people commonly call the calf muscle is actually three different muscles. These are called the gastrocnemius, the soleus, and the plantaris. The gastrocnemius raises the heel. The soleus performs the same function when the knee is in a bent position. The plantaris is responsible for rotating the ankle.

When a woman wears high heel shoes, the calves are the attractive part of the rear lower leg that catches a man's eye. For reasons that are still debated by health enthusiasts, men seem to suffer a higher incidence of calf and Achilles tendon injuries.

Since our goal as aging individuals is to optimize mobility, independence, and fitness, stretching and exercising the lower leg is something we can not afford to neglect.

As with all tendons, the Achilles tendon loses elasticity with age. Exercises that incorporate a full and natural range of motion are instrumental in helping us maintain and preserve functionality of the ankle. As was the case with upper leg exercises, we need to perform some gentle stretching of the Achilles tendon and calf muscles prior to our weight training exercises to protect against injury.

Following the stretching exercise demonstrated below, you will again select one of the suggested working exercises.

You will be performing 1 warm up set of 20 reps following by 3 working sets of 12-12-12 reps.

Notice we have made a small change to our normal number of repetitions. In the case of calves, we want to keep our repetitions slightly higher.

Variations are provided to allow you flexibility based on the equipment available to you at your facility.

Calf Stretch Raises (Warm Up Exercise)

Starting Position
Find a wooden block or other platform that allows you to stand with the balls of your feet firmly planted. Be sure the heels are able to lower as far as your natural flexibility allows without touching the floor. Grab a nearby handle or other support to help maintain your balance.

Movement
1. Slowly lower your heels off the edge of the platform. Do NOT bounce or lower your heels too rapidly. Overstretching cold, stiff Achilles tendons is a common cause of injury. Be sure to perform this stretching in a slow, steady, and full range of motion.

2. Once the heels have been lowered as far as is comfortable and you can feel the stretch in the calf muscle and tendon near the back of the heel, slowly rise up on the balls of your feet as high as possible.At the top position, you will feel the gastrocnemius muscle contract.

3. Slowly lower the heels again so they descend towards the floor in a stretched motion.

4. Repeat this motion for 20 repetitions.

5. Take a brief rest of 30 seconds. Then repeat for an additional 20 repetitions.

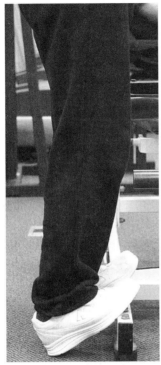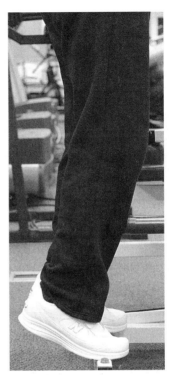

*(Photo 5.40) Calf Stretch Raises should always be performed
as a warm up prior to weight lifting exercises for the lower leg.*

Comments

Since flexibility of the Achilles tendon is so important for preventing
lower leg injuries, it can't be stressed enough that these stretching motions should be performed in a slow, steady motion.

You should really pay close attention to the amount of stretch occurring in the tendon area of the heel. This is especially important for the
first few stretches, as many people over the age of 40 have stiffness in
this area. For many people, typical daily activity and routine walking
around a home or office does not fully stretch the tendons and calf
muscles of the lower leg. For these people, injury usually results from
sudden ballistic motion like stepping off a high curb or trying to run
across the street.

With the calves and Achilles tendon now warmed up and flexible, it is time to select the working exercise for this muscle group.

Calf Machine

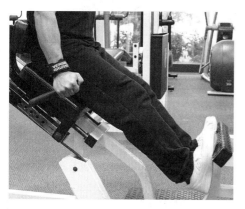 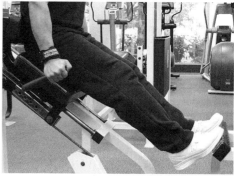

(Photo 5.41) Calf Machine

Starting Position

Adjust the sliding seat of the calf machine so that your legs are slightly bent before you begin the movement. Place the balls of your feet on the footrest. Select an appropriate weight using the selectorized weight pin. Straighten your legs until they are just shy of being totally straight. As is always the case, do NOT lock your knee joint.

When properly adjusted, you should be able to fully lower and raise the sliding seat of the machine using only your calf muscles. If you find the machine reaching its limit of travel and preventing a full range of up/down motion, try readjusting the seat.

Movement

1. Without bending your knees, rise up on the balls of your feet as high as possible. You should feel the gastrocnemius muscle contracting in this top position.

2. Once you reach the top, slowly allow the heels to descend as far as possible below your toes to get a good stretch. The overall motion

being performed here is nearly identical to the warm up exercises you just finished performing, the only difference being the addition of weighted resistance.

3. Continue this slow and steady up and down motion for the desired number of repetitions.

Comments

There are many variations of the calf machine offered by equipment manufacturers. It is a good chance you will find two or three variations of this equipment in your gym or fitness center.

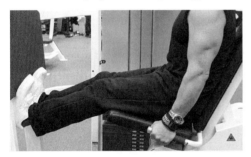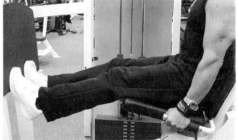

(Photo 5.42) The basic straight leg calf raise motion can be performed on several different pieces of gym equipment.

There is also a standing version of this machine that is very effective. I don't recommend the use of the standing version for older individuals since it requires supporting moderate to heavy weights on the shoulders as you perform the lowering and raising motion. Since lower back and spinal problems are very common for older individuals, I tend to steer clear of exercise motions that apply a large downward pressure on the spinal column.

Joint protection while strengthening muscles is a priority for those of us over 50. Any exercise that places a large downward force on the spine may potentially contribute to compression of the intervertebral discs or aggravation of that condition if it already exists.

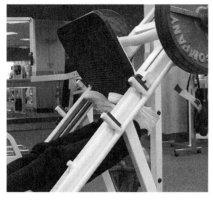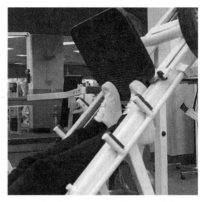

(Photo 5.43) Yet another variation on the basic weighted calf raise motion.

To summarize, while the standing calf raise is excellent for working the gastrocnemius, we have many options available to us that work those muscles equally well without placing strain on the back and spine.

Seated Calf Raises

Starting Position
Load the machine with an appropriate number of plates. Sit down on the machine seat and place the balls of your feet on the foot bar. Your heels should be suspended. Adjust the length of the column on the knee pad so that the pads wedge snugly over your knees. When properly adjusted, the machine will allow for a full range of upper and lower motion without reaching the end of its travel.

Movement
1. With your lower legs tense and ready to accept the weight, reach forward and release the stop bar.

2. Slowly lower the weight by bending the ankles and allowing the heels to lower towards the floor. Do not bounce or descend too quickly.

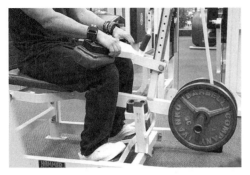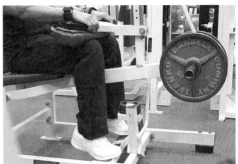

(Photo 5.44) Seated Calf Raises

3. When you have reached the lowest point you can comfortably go, and you feel a good stretch in your calves, slowly and firmly raise your heels so that you end up with your heels high in the air with the weight supported on the balls of your feet.

4. Repeat this motion for the desired number of repetitions.

Comments

The basic up/down movement of the heels during seated calf raises is the same as that performed on the calf machine. However, as similar as they may seem, these exercises focus on different parts of the lower leg.

As mentioned earlier, when heels are raised from a straight leg position, the gastrocnemius muscle does most of the work. Conversely, when the same heel raising motion is done with a bent leg, the soleus muscle assumes most of the workload.

In order to fully exercise the calf muscles, it is highly recommended that you routinely alternate between these two different exercises. One day you might perform the standard calf machine with a straight leg. During your next visit to the gym, you should do the seated version.

With the completion of the calf exercises, we have reached the end of our weight resistance training.

We will now move our focus to the waist and midsection.

MIDSECTION

Very few people today, much less those of us in our 50s, are happy with our waist and midsection.

Middle age spread seems more common today than sand on a beach. As we discussed earlier, the real "secret" behind a trim and firm waist is diet. An overweight person can perform 1,000 sit-ups per day for the remainder of their lives, or invest in every type of tummy shaper advertised on late night TV, with no visible results.

There is an old saying, "You can't flex fat." The message here is no matter how firm the stomach may be, it will never be visible if it is hidden under a blanket of excess fat. Sit-ups and any other form of abdominal exercise will strengthen the muscles of the midsection, but they will not "burn" away the fat in that region.

It is also important to remember that excess body fat accumulates from the inside out. This means if you can "pinch more than an inch" or otherwise feel you look overweight around the middle, then you already have substantial excess body fat inside your body surrounding your organs.

Let me reiterate this fact one more time: Diet is crucial for losing excess body weight. With this fact in mind, let's continue our discussion of the midsection.

In recent years, the concept of training your body's core has become a popular trend. In essence, the idea here is to strengthen the entire region of the body that helps stabilize the spine and pelvis. As an aging individual, we have similar goals. When we design an exercise regimen for our midsection, we are not only focused on the abdominal muscles but also the lower back, lower pelvic region, and lateral sides of the waist.

Exercising the midsection for people over 40 is intended to strengthen the entire region to help improve posture, maintain flexibility, minimize risks of hernia, and reduce problems associated with lower back pain.

Our regimen for exercising the midsection will be a bit different than what we did for other body parts. In this case we will be performing a few different exercises.

You will perform one set of each exercise in succession. The goal is to perform 20 repetitions of each exercise, although it is to be expected that some people will only be able to perform half that many at the beginning. That is OK. We are trying to improve ourselves here. If you were already in perfect shape for your age, it is a good chance you would not be reading this book.

People already plagued with a history of lower back problems should consult their doctor before performing most of these exercises. While all the movements shown here are time-tested and well documented as excellent exercises for training the midsection, it is possible that certain individuals may have unique spinal problems that could be aggravated by repetitive waist motion.

So, if you have no serious back problems, and your personal physician agrees you can benefit from the program described in these chapters, let's get to work on that midsection.

Crunches

Starting Position

Lie on your back with your heels resting on the surface of a bench or other flat surface. The height of this support should be such that your thighs are perpendicular to the floor. Your knees should be in an approximate 90 degree angle.

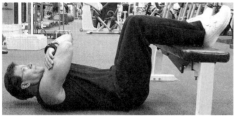
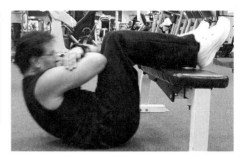

(Photo 5.45) Crunches

Cross your arms in front of your chest or at the sides of your head. (see Photos 5.45 and 5.46)

Movement

1. Earlier we discussed proper breathing techniques when exerting force to lift a weight. That wisdom also comes into play when exercising the midsection. When training the waist, we want to avoid building up intrathoracic pressure inside the abdomen. This is achieved by remembering to exhale when crunching forward and inhaling when lying backwards.

2. Keeping this breathing rhythm in mind, slightly raise your hips off the floor, suck in your stomach slightly, while at the same time curling (crunching) your upper body forward towards your knees, effectively shortening your torso.

3. Be sure to exhale during this entire forward motion while feeling the contraction in your whole abdominal region.

Comments

The crunch replaces the common sit up most of us did back in school. Since that time, several studies have revealed that the traditional sit up is not as effective as the crunch for targeting the abdominal region. In fact, the common sit up shifts much of the work to the hip flexors and can also aggravate lower back pain.

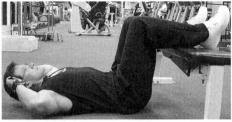
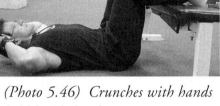
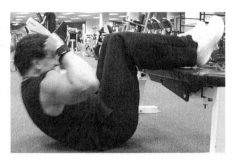

(Photo 5.46) Crunches with hands held beside head

The crunch looks like a simple exercise with a small range of motion, but it is actually a bit tricky to perform properly. In order to be totally effective, you must simultaneously raise the hips slightly, exhale your breath, curl your body forward, and vacuum your waist in slightly.

Don't think of sitting up as much as curling your upper body forward like those small worms you sometimes see in the garden in the spring time. You may need to experiment a little with the timing of your small hip lift, breathing, sucking your stomach in, and curling forward—but once you do the motion properly and feel your abdominals doing all the work, you will never forget the feeling.

People often remark they only feel tension in their upper abdominals when they do crunches. When performed as described above, you will feel the entire abdominal region contributing to the effort. You will then have mastered the crunch.

Leg Raises

Starting Position
Lie on your back on the floor. Form a triangle-shaped cradle with your hands and place them beneath your buttocks to offer lower back support. Extend your legs straight out with your knees only slightly bent.

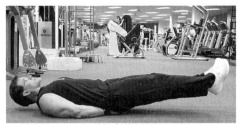

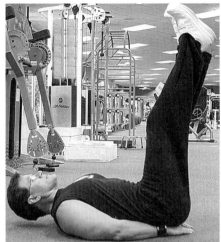

(Photo 5.47) Leg Raises

Movement

1. While exhaling, slowly raise your legs using your lower abdominal muscles until they are not quite perpendicular to the ground.

2. While inhaling, slowly lower your legs until your heels are just 1–2" off the floor. Do not allow your heels to touch the floor.

3. Once again slowly raise your legs to the top position.

4. Repeat this movement for the desired number of repetitions.

Comments

In the movement description for this exercise, you will notice it mentioned that your heels should not touch the floor at any time during your repetitions. Additionally, we stress not letting your legs rise all the way to a 90 degree angle. The goal is to keep tension on the lower abdominals during the full movement and duration of the exercise. Resting the heels on the floor or raising the legs until they are at a perfect 90 degree angle will take the workload off the abdominals.

Toning the lower abdominals is important but often neglected by many people who only focus on doing sit up motions. In fact, most people experience weakness and sagging of the lower abdominals with age. The lower abdominal region around the navel is where many people complain they first notice "belly bulge."

Hyperextensions for Lower Back

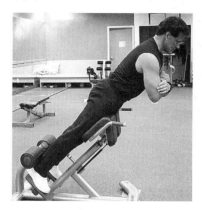
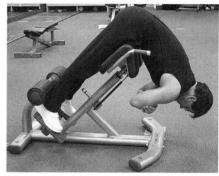

(Photo 5.48) Hyperextensions for the lower back

Starting Position

I want to make a special cautionary note that people with a history of lower back or disc problems should consult their doctor before performing this exercise.

Lie facedown on the hyperextension bench. Secure your ankles under the support pads. Lean forward such that your upper thighs rest on the main padding. Be sure the pad is not too high. Your waist should be able to freely bend forward from the hips. You should not be placing any pressure on the lower abdomen or laying on your stomach in any way. You should only feel your weight being supported by the upper thighs. Cross your arms in front of your chest.

Movement

1. While exhaling, slowly bend forward at the waist as far as you can while keeping a slight arch in your back. Your back should not be bowed during this movement. At the bottom position, you will be suspended with your head near the floor.

2. Once you have reached the bottom, slowly raise your upper body until the legs and torso form a straight line similar to when you are in a standing position. Do NOT exaggerate the upwards movement by raising yourself too far into a backwards bend. You want to bend fully forward, but only rise to a straight position. You should feel the work being performed by your lower back. You may also feel the hamstrings of the rear leg contributing to the effort.

3. Beginners may not be able to complete the desired number of repetitions of this exercise at one time. Start with as many as you can do using proper form and work up to the desired number of repetitions.

Comments

The Hyperextension is an excellent exercise to strengthen and improve stability in the lower back. This movement directly works the spinal erectors, with secondary benefit extending to the glutes and hamstrings.

For many people who suffer occasional back problems, but have no diagnosed spinal or disc damage, the cause is often a weakness in the spinal erector muscles. As the name implies, the spinal erectors primarily function to extend your torso. They also allow you to straighten up when leaning forward. When contracting, these muscles assist in keeping your torso stable.

Often times when somebody says "my back went out," they may not have any actual structural flaw in the vertebrae or discs but are probably experiencing a fatigue in the spinal erectors.

When I was in my 30s, I went through a period of many years where I was not eating properly or exercising regularly. I was working seven days a week, 12–16 hours per day trying to build a new business with some partners. It was the typical tough entrepreneurial business start–up. During times like this, we sometimes fail to take care of ourselves as we throw everything we have into the venture.

One day, a chair broke as I was sitting down. I hit the floor with a force that sent a jolting pain shooting through my lower back. For the next few years, whenever I would do yard work or other extended physical activity I would get to the point where I could hardly stand up straight. At times, the pain was so bad I would be on my knees on the floor. On other occasions, I was just trying to find a comfortable way to lie on the floor to rest my back.

The doctors confirmed that I had no serious damage, yet the problem with back pain and frequent weakness continued. Around that time I heard about hyperextensions being used by physical therapists and professional boxers as a way to strengthen the lower back. I started doing this movement several times per week in an attempt to rehabilitate and strengthen my own lower back. I have continued performing this motion 2–3 times per week over the years.

Today, 20 years later, I have no lower back problems and actually feel better than I did in 1993. I can spend a whole day pushing a wheel barrow around the yard laying sod and bags of mulch on a one acre property and have no lower back discomfort. As a younger man two decades ago, that kind of heavy duty yard work would have left me crippled and hurting for several days.

To summarize: the hyperextension is a great exercise to strengthen the spinal erectors and may help you avoid ever facing lower back problems. For those people who already suffer from lower back issues, this movement may be beneficial in diminishing discomfort and restoring functionality.

But again, due to the unique medical histories we all live with, you should discuss with your doctor if this exercise is a good idea for your personal condition.

Congratulations, you have just finished the weight resistance and mid-section portion of the 30-3 Routine. You have exercised all the major muscle groups as well as your abdominal and lower back region.

Now it is time to perform the cardiovascular part of your regimen. Grab your water bottle, towel, and portable MP3 player and let's head over to the cardio section of your gym.

The 30-3 Cardiovascular Exercise Details

As you may have ascertained by now, the 3 in our 30-3 Routine name refers to the number of working sets we routinely perform for each muscle group. It also refers to the number of days per week you perform this routine.

Now we address the 30. Immediately following weight training, we next perform 30 minutes of cardiovascular exercise.

You may be asking the question, "Why do we do the cardio after the weight training. Why don't we do the cardio first?" There are two closely related reasons to perform weight training prior to cardio.

First, when we begin our routine, we are rested and our muscles are full of glycogen. This allows you to exert more force and strength in your lifts. This maximizes the benefit of weight resistance training.

Secondly, a majority of people are concerned with weight loss. If we first burn excess glycogen reserves by forcing the muscles to lift weights, we begin our cardio session better able to start burning excess fat. As you will recall from our chapter on diet, nutrition, and weight loss, once the body has no excess carbohydrates or glycogen reserves available to use for energy, it must start utilizing fat to derive the energy it needs. That is how you truly lose weight in the form of excess body fat.

Our goal as an older individual is to build up healthy endurance and maintain at least 30 minutes of cardiovascular (cardio) activity during each session.

Just as was the case with weight resistance training, you are strongly advised to discuss cardiovascular exercise with your doctor. As mentioned previously, it is impossible to know the unique medical histories of every reader. While the advice and tips offered here are well researched and have been effective for numerous people, you may have a special ailment, illness, or injury that will require special consideration. I invite you to share the diet and exercise routines described in this book with your personal physician to ensure that they are 100% suitable to your needs.

How Much Cardio Should I Do?

Your goal will be to build up to 30 minutes.

Depending on your current level of fitness, 30 minutes of continuous cardio activity may be too demanding at first. If this is the case, start with a shorter time interval of 10–15 minutes, or whatever you can handle.

But wait a minute you say—30 minutes is only a time duration. How intense should the 30 minutes of cardio exercise be? 30 minutes of casually strolling around the block is far different than jogging for half an hour.

In order to increase cardiovascular fitness and burn fat, you need to exercise within your Target Heart Rate.

What is the Target Heart Rate (THR)?

Medical researchers have established that in order to gain significant benefit from any cardiovascular related exercise, the heart rate must be elevated to a higher than normal level for at least 20 minutes.

Different sources will show some minor deviation in the upper and lower limits for suggested THR, but they are all essentially in the same ball park.

The first step in knowing your Target Heart Rate range is to calculate your Maximum Heart Rate in beats per minute. Maximum heart rate is calculated using the formula:

Maximum Heart Rate (bpm) = 220 – Your Age

Example: For a 50 year old individual.
MHR = 220 – 50 = 170 bpm

The Mayo Foundation for Medical Education and Research as well as the Center for Disease Control and Prevention utilize the values of 70% MHR and 85% MHR to determine the range you should aim for when performing vigorous cardiovascular exercise.

The CDC, as well as fitness professionals who work with rehabilitation patients and the elderly, will often aim for a milder Target Heart Range of 50% MHR to 70% MHR. This range is also desirable when working with individuals new to an exercise routine or having prior health concerns.

Continuing with our example for a 50 year old individual:

Moderate Activity Target Heart Range (50-70% of MHR)
Lower Rate Limit (bpm) = MHR x 0.50
Upper Rate Limit (bpm) = MHR x 0.70

Example: For our 50 year old test subject.
Lower Rate Limit = 170 x 0.50 = 85 bpm
Upper Rate Limit = 170 x 0.70 = 119 bpm

Vigorous Activity Target Heart Range (70-85% of MHR)

Lower Rate Limit (bpm) = MHR x 0.70
Upper Rate Limit (bpm) = MHR x 0.85

Example: For our 50 year old test subject.
Lower Rate Limit = 170 x 0.70 = 119 bpm
Upper Rate Limit = 170 x 0.85 = 145 bpm

In the example above, we can see that a 50-year-old person aiming to perform 30 minutes of cardio exercise at a moderate intensity level should keep their heart rate between 85–119 beats per minute.

The same individual who is better conditioned, and free of any known medical conditions, may wish to perform at a more vigorous level. In this case, they would aim to maintain their heart rate between 119–145 for the full 30 minutes of cardio exercise.

The Maximum Heart Rate and subsequent target ranges are all derived from an empirical formula derived through years of research by medical professionals. While history has shown this calculation to be very accurate for the vast majority of people, it is very important that you discuss your personal health conditions with your doctor. There are a variety of medical conditions, as well as medications (such as beta blockers), that are known to have an effect on maximum heart rate.

You now know what Target Heart Range is and how it is calculated. You also understand that these theoretical ranges may need to be slightly adjusted based on your personal medical history. A personal physician can offer some guidance in regard to this issue.

For your convenience, the chart below shows these MHR and THR values for ages 30 through 105, calculated at five year intervals.

Age	Max Heart Rate-bpm	50% MHR	70% MHR	85% MHR
30	190	95	133	162
35	185	93	130	157
40	180	90	126	153
45	175	88	123	149
50	170	85	119	145
55	165	83	116	140
60	160	80	112	136
65	155	78	109	132
70	150	75	105	128
75	145	73	102	123
80	140	70	98	119
85	135	68	95	115
90	130	65	91	111
95	125	63	88	106
100	120	60	84	102
105	115	58	81	98

Example of Chart Usage:
If our 50-year-old test subject is given a green light by their doctor to perform cardiovascular exercise *(most doctors will encourage cardio if no special medical conditions exist)*, then it may be appropriate to stay in the 50%–70% range of 85–119 bpm for the first few months.

This is especially advisable if a person has not exercised regularly for several years. Gradually, as the level of fitness improves, our 50–year–old test subject should aim to perform cardiovascular exercise in the 70%–85% range of 119–145 bpm.

Equipment Options

Gyms today offer a vast array of cardio equipment. Chances are good if you are at a gym or hospital fitness center of any reasonable size you will see treadmills, ellipticals, stair machines, bicycles, and rowing machines, among others.

Each of these pieces of equipment will provide you with a good cardio workout, but at this stage we are going to limit ourselves to two of the more popular —treadmill and elliptical. Both the treadmill and elliptical are easy on the knees and adapt to virtually any stride length, making it comfortable to perform for the desired 30 minutes.

Treadmills can be used at a flat setting with a rapid walking speed, or set to an incline of as much as 20 degrees for more of an uphill feeling of intensity. Women especially like using the treadmill on a steep slope with a long stride as it helps to shape and round the buttocks.

The elliptical machine offers the extra benefit of giving your arms and chest a small workout in addition to the primary cardiovascular and legs benefit.

Knee joint health is always a concern for older individuals. For that reason, I shy away from recommending the various stair climbing cardio machines for people over the age of 50. Stair climbing will certainly give you an intense cardio workout, but for many individuals, these machines can cause knee discomfort.

By the very nature of their design, most of these machines have a fixed step size that rotates like an endless stationary staircase. The problem for some individuals is these step sizes do not match their normal stride length. In an attempt to change their length of stride and leg angle to match the rotating stair steps, some people experience an awkward feeling in their knees and hips.

I am one of those people. In real life I rarely walk up stairs one step at a time. I routinely use every other step when walking up a stairwell. This is simply where my legs naturally want to go. Using every step often feels choppy, like I am cutting short each forward motion of my leg.

I have used various makes of stair climbers over the years, and only two were comfortable for me to use. On most of the others, I would experience discomfort in my knees and hips in only 2–3 minutes —long before I even started to get the least bit winded. I have spoken to others who express this same experience.

But by the same token, there are hundreds of thousands of people who use these machines daily with no complaints whatsoever. It is my opinion that the variability lies in the individual. Unlike something like a free weight dumbbell which can move in perfect harmony with your body's size and shape and joint angles, ANY type of exercise equipment has limited sizing options.

This is especially true of the stair climbing exercisers which feature one size and step height. If by chance you are the perfect size and have a natural stride length that meshes with the machine, you are probably going to love it. By contrast, a particularly short- or long-limbed individual may experience the awkwardness and joint issues discussed above.

I certainly encourage you to try these cardio exercisers and see if they are for you. I don't want to discourage the use of a machine that may be beneficial in helping you to realize your fitness goals. I only want to make you aware that by nature of their design, the treadmill and elliptical are more comfortable and natural feeling. They easily accommodate people of all sizes and stride lengths.

With a variety of angles and intensities available, both of these machines can also be set to provide more than sufficient stimulus to allow you to exercise inside your target heart rate range.

Treadmill

Using the treadmill is as simple as walking. Some people may be inclined to ask the question, "Why is a treadmill any more beneficial than
walking around my neighborhood?" This is a fair question. In fact, there
are a number of advantages offered by the treadmill that don't always
immediately come to mind.

- Despite the best of intentions, it is often hard to maintain a fast
  walking pace when simply taking a walk around your block or
  through the park. All too often our minds begin to think about
  other issues in our lives and before we realize it, we have slowed our
  walking speed down considerably. In this regard, the treadmill helps
  us by maintaining a set speed.

- Treadmills allow for variable resistance by offering inclines typically ranging from flat to 15 degrees. These different slopes not only
  change intensity but also target different walking muscles. A steep
  incline impacts your buttocks,
  calves, and hamstrings more than
  walking flat. These inclines are
  especially useful for people living
  in flat terrain regions such as the
  Midwestern Plains and Florida
  where natural hills do not exist.

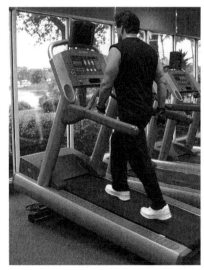

- Treadmills offer the ability to walk
  in any climate condition. Regardless of the outside weather being
  rainy, cold, hot, or covered in
  snow, you can always jump on the
  treadmill.

- For those who simply can't
  stand to miss their favorite TV

*(Photo 5.49) Treadmill. In this
example, incline is set to 15 degrees and speed is 2.5 mph.*

show but are exercising on a tight schedule, most gyms now have treadmills equipped with individual TV screens. These equipment-mounted TV screens also feature earphone jacks so you can watch your program of choice without external distractions.

- Most modern treadmills feature the ability to give real time readings of your heart rate. This makes it easy to stay within your target range throughout your workout. In fact, virtually all modern treadmills feature preset programs that offer variety in intensity. Additionally, as an aid to keeping track of your progress, they also provide information such as total distance walked and calories burned.

Starting Position

Stand on the treadmill. Most of these machines prompt you for weight and time and perhaps other variables such as the type of walk you desire to perform. These options normally range from simple manual control of incline and speed to preprogrammed trails that emulate random walks up hills, through mountains, etc.

The first few times you start using the treadmill, it may be wise to select the manual setting where you can fully control the speed and incline as needed to maintain your target heart range. As you improve both in fitness level and gain a familiarity of the machine, you can try the random programmed settings.

Movement

1. Simply walk at a brisk pace with a full natural stride.

2. Periodically use the sensors provided to monitor your heart rate and ensure you are inside your target zone.

3. Depending on your comfort level, you may either swing arms freely as when everyday walking, or place a light hold on one of the support rails for balance.

4. As needed, adjust the incline and speed of the treadmill so that you remain inside your Target Heart Rate zone for 30 minutes.

Comments

In your earliest stages of walking on the treadmill, you may choose to select a fixed incline and speed which provides suitable resistance to keep you in your target heart rate range. *(For example, a 9 degree incline and speed of 3.3 mph is about right for me.)*

However, recent research has shown additional benefit is derived when the work intensity is variable over time as opposed to being a static condition. This means that instead of spending the full 30 minutes walking at an incline of 9 degrees and a speed of 3.3 and maintaining a heart rate of 130bpm, our 50-year-old test subject may periodically change the speed and incline to offer variable resistance and heart rate.

For 5 minutes, a shallow incline and quicker walking speed of 4.0 mph may be selected. Then for the next 5 minutes, the incline is ramped up to 15 degrees and the speed lowered to 2.5 mph. This type of incline and speed change can be used every 5 minutes or so to introduce variability.

During these types of changes the heart rate will of course increase and decrease to meet the demand. The important thing is to be sure you stay between the lower and upper limits of your target zone. In this example, with our 50-year-old who may be aiming for a vigorous training level, his heart rate will fluctuate between 119–145bpm throughout the 30 minute routine.

An additional benefit of this variability is that it places emphasis on different leg muscles. It will also minimize joint discomfort which sometimes occurs from repetitive identical motion.

Elliptical

Some people feel the elliptical to be an ideal machine for cardiovascular fitness. Unlike the treadmill or stationary bike, an elliptical machine features movable arms that work similar to ski poles. As you run or walk on the elliptical machine, these arms allow you to involve your upper body muscles in the workout.

Utilizing more muscles while you exercise helps burn more calories. The extra upper body motion helps tone arms and shoulders at the same time. Elliptical machines also offer a number of other positive features:

- By the very nature of their design, elliptical machines are less stressful on your bones and joints.

- Most modern commercial elliptical machines feature built-in heart rate monitors. They also track your speed, intensity, time, distance traveled, and total calories burned.

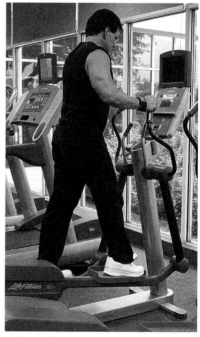

- Elliptical machines often feature built-in TV screens with private speaker jacks, a cooling fan, plus different preset workouts that offer variety and variable resistance.

- A common practice you will see on elliptical machines is people striding backwards. When you reverse stride, you work your quadriceps, hamstrings, glutes, and calves in a different way. This movement is also beneficial for those trying to improve balance and coordination. When going from forward motion to backward, you should first come to a

(Photo 5.50) Elliptical

full stop. Then focus your weight onto the back of your legs. Keep a straight posture when moving backward. Using the moveable arms for support is even more important for walking backwards than it is for the standard forward motion.

Starting Position

Stand on the elliptical machine. The pedals on these machines are quite large, allowing you to position your feet where the stride is most comfortable.

Most of these machines prompt you for weight and time, and perhaps other variables such as the type of intensity you desire to perform. The first few times you start using the elliptical, it may be wise to select the manual setting where you can control the intensity to maintain your target heart range. As you improve both in fitness level and gain a familiarity with the machine, you can try the random programmed settings.

Grasp the handles of the moveable arms at a height that will simulate the motion of cross country skiing when in motion.

Movement

1. The best way to describe the motion of the elliptical machine is being nearly identical to cross country skiing. With your feet remaining planted in position, begin a forward skiing motion.

2. You can increase the benefit to your arms and shoulder and chest by applying push and pull pressure on the moveable handles while in motion.

3. Monitor your heart rate and fine tune the combination of intensity level and speed that allows you to remain inside your Target Heart Rate zone for 30 minutes.

Comments

If you do not suffer from any lower back or spinal problems, you may wish to experiment with letting your waist slightly rotate as you perform this movement. Done properly, you should feel your oblique muscles along the sides of the waist get involved from this mild twisting motion. After all, who doesn't want to firm up the love handles a bit more? A combination of healthy diet and a gentle bit of twisting on the elliptical while performing cardio can really tighten up the midsection.

Measuring Heart Rate

Thus far we have assumed the cardio machines of your choice will feature heart rate monitors. Today this is a fair assumption since it has pretty much become industry standard. Despite this fact, there may be times when the monitor is broken, or, the facility you visit has older equipment. If this is the case, you can measure your heart rate the good old-fashioned way.

To manually check your heart rate, place your index and middle fingers together on the opposite wrist, about 1/2 inch on the inside of the joint, in line with the index finger. Once you find a pulse, count the number of beats you feel within a one minute period.

A shortcut to this procedure is to count the number of beats in a 15 second span of time and multiply by 4. The shortcut method is prone to be a bit less accurate since you are extrapolating a result from a brief measured time interval.

Another suggestion that is recommended for those getting serious about fitness is a heart rate monitor. At the time of this writing, small reliable heart rate monitors no larger than a wristwatch are available for $30–40. These can be found at almost any sporting goods store or conveniently purchased online from popular sites such as Amazon.com.

Hey You Did It

You have just finished a full 30-3 Routine, composed of weight resistance training and cardiovascular exercise. In 12–16 weeks, combined with the diet principles you learned earlier, you will see and feel significant improvement in your overall fitness and energy.

Now, for the sake of convenience, on the following page you'll find a summary of the 30-3 Routine you can copy and carry with you for reference until you have it memorized.

30-3 Routine Quick Reference Guide

Perform 5-minute Warm Up routine before beginning training.
Unless otherwise noted, select one exercise for each body part.
Perform 1 Warm Up Set of 20 reps + 3 Working Sets of 12-10-8 reps.

Chest
Incline Barbell Press OR Incline Dumbbell Press

Shoulders
Machine Shoulder Press OR Dumbbell Shoulder Press

Triceps
Triceps Pulley Pushdowns OR Triceps Extension Machine

Back
Seated Pulley OR Seated Machine Rows OR Lat Pull downs

Biceps
Barbell Curl OR Cambered Bar Curls OR Dumbbell Curls

Quadriceps (front of leg)
Leg Extensions (3 warm up sets) prior to primary exercise.
Angled Leg Press OR Seated Leg Press

Hamstrings (back of leg)
Lying Leg Curl OR Seated Leg Curl

Calves
Calf Stretch Raises (2 warm up sets) prior to primary exercise.
Calf Machine OR Seated Calf Raises
Warm Up Set of 20 reps + 3 Working Sets of 12-12-12 reps

Midsection
Crunches and Leg Raises and Lower Back Hyperextensions
1 set of 20 reps for each exercise

Cardio
Treadmill OR Elliptical Machine
30 minutes in Target Heart Range

Chapter Six

Taking It to the Next Level
3 Day per Week Split Routine

Congratulations, if you are reading these words, you are ready to move up to the next step in your fitness program.

At this stage, you have spent at least 8–12 weeks performing the 30-3 Routine and should be feeling improvements in your overall fitness and energy. As you neared the 12 week mark, you should have also started seeing significant improvements in the mirror.

I also hope you have had a chance to discuss the fitness ideas in this book with your doctor to ensure that they are compatible with your personal history and current health condition.

With foundation training completed, you are now ready to achieve some super results. The routine to be discussed in this chapter essentially establishes the regimen you will follow for the remainder of your years on planet Earth.

Now, let's take it to another level.

The 3 Day per Week Split Routine

The full body routine you have been doing until now is an excellent and very effective regimen for generally conditioning the body. It is especially helpful in creating a foundation of fitness for those who have not participated in any form of regular exercise for some time. It is also a routine that some doctors may advise elderly patients to maintain in later years.

However, for the majority of people aged 40–70, the 30-3 routine alone is unable to provide the full stimulation our older bodies require to best offset the effects of aging. Once an 8–12 week baseline level of fitness is established, our exercise routine must be a bit more scientifically structured to provide optimum intensity for each major muscle group while also providing sufficient time for rest and recuperation.

In order to accomplish this goal, you will no longer be exercising the full body each time you go to the gym. Instead we are going to split the body into three sections. We will focus only on those sections (or groups) each of the three days we go to the gym. In this way, each of your three weekly visits to the gym will be totally different.

By splitting the body into groups, we are able to incorporate more movements, more sets, and more reps for each of the body parts in a given training session. This increased intensity and time under tension provides more stimulation for the muscle to firm and strengthen.

Split routines are common among bodybuilders and pro athletes. We have simply taken this knowledge and time proven technique and adapted it to our specific needs.

This routine includes the following basic features:
- Body is divided into 3 groups
- Each group is exercised 1 day per week
- 3 total visits to the gym each week
- 2 to 3 different exercises performed per body part

- Most exercises generally follow our 3 sets of 12-10-8 reps rule
- Each major body part is trained with a total of 6–9 working sets
- 30 minutes of cardiovascular training

Although this may seem a bit complex at first, it is really just an expansion of what you have already been doing. Instead of working your entire body on the same day with only one exercise for each body part, you are splitting your body up over three days and doing two or three different exercises for each body part.

Following are the details of the weight training regimen, descriptions of the exercises, and options for the cardiovascular portion of your training.

At the end of the chapter, I will use the guidelines described below to create a sample training program you can use as a model to customize your own favorite routines.

The 3 Day Split Routine Weight Resistance Training Details

Your body will be divided into three groups. Each day you go to the gym, you will work on only that group. You will normally be performing three different exercises for each body part in that day's group.

You will begin by doing a warm up set of 15–20 repetitions with a light weight just as you performed in your earlier workouts. The purpose of this set is to get the muscles, joints, and connective tissue warmed up and acclimated to the range of motion before being subjected to a working load.

Afterwards, you will usually perform three working sets of 12 reps, then 10 reps, then 8 reps.

There are a few exceptions to these general guidelines that will be detailed in the applicable section.

You should increase the weight slightly every time you move to a set with lower repetitions. For example, a good chest training portion of the regimen may look like this:

Incline Dumbbell Press:

Warm-up Set	20 pounds	20 reps
Working Set 1	35 pounds	12 reps
Working Set 2	45 pounds	10 reps
Working Set 3	60 pounds	8 reps

Flat Barbell Press:

Warm-up Set	45 pounds	20 reps
Working Set 1	75 pounds	12 reps
Working Set 2	90 pounds	10 reps
Working Set 3	125 pounds	8 reps

Incline Dumbbell Fly:

Warm-up Set	12 pounds	20 reps
Working Set 1	20 pounds	12 reps
Working Set 2	25 pounds	10 reps
Working Set 3	35 pounds	8 reps

You will then move immediately to the next body part in that day's group.

Remember the rule for selecting the proper amount of weight: select an amount that allows you to just barely complete the desired number of reps before reaching a point of near failure.

In the example above, when performing Working Set 3 for 8 repetitions, you should just barely be able to complete the final repetition using proper form. The idea of trying to continue onward with 12 or more reps should seem very difficult, if not impossible. However, if you easily zip through all the working sets and have not needed to exert some effort to finish the last 1–2 reps in each set, then you are using too little weight.

Grouping the Body Parts

When dividing the body into sections, we don't simply do so randomly. The groups are formulated based on physiology and logic. There are a few points to consider:

- Large muscle groups require more energy to train. In order to be able to endure a full workout, only one large muscle group should be worked per day.

- Our objective is optimized benefit with minimal wear and tear on joints, ligaments, and tendons. Therefore, sufficient rest is needed between exercising overlapping body parts.

- As aging individuals, we are more concerned with functional mobility as opposed to a specialized sports function.

Referring to the points above, the three largest muscle groups of the body are Chest, Quadriceps, and Back. We want to work these different large muscle groups on separate days.

When selecting smaller muscle groups to be performed along with these larger groups, it is functionally beneficial to work the body in "Push-Pull" groupings.

This means on one day, you primarily work the muscles of your body that push. The next time you train, you work the muscles that pull. As an example of this point, think of your arm. The biceps on the front of your arm is a pulling muscle. By contrast, the triceps on the back of the arm is engaged whenever you are pushing something away from you.

Taking all the above points into consideration, we will be splitting our body into the following three groups:

- Chest, Shoulders, Triceps
- Quadriceps, Hamstrings, Calves
- Back, Biceps, Trapezius, Forearms

Cardio and exercises for the midsection will be performed with each group.

First, Second, and Third Exercise Movements
For most of the body parts, we are going to incorporate a basic power movement as our first exercise. This will then be followed by one or two other complimentary exercises that work that same muscle group from different angles and recruit additional fibers.

Why do we make this distinction? Some exercises are very effective at working the majority of a muscle group. These serve as a "bread and butter" movement. These kinds of exercises normally allow you to use heavier weights and incorporate considerable power into the movement.

By comparison, other exercises are sometimes more effective at refining or simply toning the muscles. Exercise professionals refer to these as either compound or isolation exercises.

It is no coincidence that compound movements were used in the 30-3 routine to build a solid foundation for fitness. In order to obtain maximum benefit from your exercise routine, you must be sure to incorporate both compound and isolation movements in each workout. Some people make the mistake of avoiding basic compound movements and only perform isolation exercises. These individuals often end up disappointed by a lack of results.

In order to help you avoid making this same mistake, I will be dividing the exercise options for each body part into categories. You simply need to select one exercise from each category to ensure that you are incorporating both compound and isolation movements. This variety of exercises will ensure that you fully work each muscle group.

I'll next describe the exercises for each body part themselves. For most of the exercises, I have included alternatives of the same basic movement. These alternatives are useful since they allow you to incorporate variety into your routine. Having options also allows you to adapt your workouts in case the gym is busy, or certain pictured equipment is not available at your facility. As mentioned earlier, it is always a good idea to incorporate variety in your routine every few weeks. Do not always select the same three exercises for months or years on end.

Additionally, all the tips you learned earlier regarding full and natural range of motion, hand positioning, and proper breathing are still applicable in this training regimen. Those basic principles are always important to keep in mind when performing any kind of exercise motion.

Great care has been taken in creating the different categories for each body part. If you follow the simple rule of choosing one exercise from each category, you can't go wrong.

Let's get started with the first of your three workouts for the upcoming week.

Day 1: Chest, Shoulders, Triceps

The chest, shoulders, and triceps work in combination to form the primary pushing force of your upper body. When pushing, these three major muscle groups work together to varying degrees. The contribution of each muscle group to the overall effort will change depending upon the angle of motion. Lifting a tree limb over your head will use more shoulder strength, while pushing a car will require more effort from your chest and triceps.

By working these upper body pushing muscles together on the same day, you will not only increase your overall strength, but also improve coordination.

WARM-UP

Prior to beginning the weight resistance training for the day, perform the 5 minute warm up routine we discussed in the last chapter.

CHEST

As with most of the body parts that follow, we are going to incorporate a basic power movement as our first exercise when working the chest. This will then be followed up with an exercise chosen from each of the two subsequent lists.

First Exercise Movement
Incline Barbell Press
Incline Dumbbell Press

Second Exercise Movement
Flat Barbell Bench Press
Flat Dumbbell Press
Seated Chest Press Machine

Third Exercise Movement
Seated Pec Machine
Dumbbell Flyes
Cable Crossovers

Choose **one** exercise from each of the lists above.

For each exercise, perform 1 warm up set of 20 reps followed by 3 working sets of 12-10-8 reps.

The detailed description and photo demonstration for each exercise are as follows:

Incline Barbell Press (described in previous chapter)

Incline Dumbbell Press (described in previous chapter)

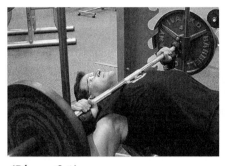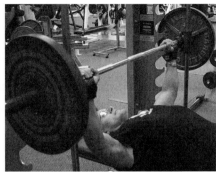

(Photo 6.1)
Flat Barbell Bench Press on 3D Motion Smith Press Machine

Flat Barbell Press

Starting Position
Lay on a flat horizontal bench. Reach up and grab the bar approximately 3–5 inches wider than your shoulders. Keep your shoulders back with your chest forward. Keep your feet planted firmly on the floor for support.

Movement
1. Remove the bar from the supports with a small lifting motion.

2. Lower the weight in a controlled motion so that the bar just barely touches your chest in the general region of the nipple line. Your upper arms should be at almost right angles to your torso.

3. Straighten your arms with a slight accelerated force so that the weight is pressed upward along the same arc to the starting position. Do NOT lock out your elbows. Be sure your shoulders remain pulled back during the full motion.

4. Repeat for the desired number of repetitions.

Comments

The flat bench press is considered one of the most basic movements for the pectorals and a top exercise for overall upper body development.

During the motion, your forearms should be in a perpendicular position under the bar, with the elbows staying under the wrists. If you notice that your wrists are flared inwards or outwards at an angle, your hand position is either too narrow or too wide.

As was the case when describing incline presses, a common mistake made by many is pushing the bar too high. When the shoulders are arched higher than the chest, the chest tends to cave in and the front shoulder muscles begin doing all the work. This is an undesirable scenario.

The shoulders should always remain pulled back behind the chest, and the chest muscles should be where you feel the work being performed. In the demonstration photo (Photo 6.1), a free motion form of Smith Machine is being used. This equipment offers both 3D motion and safety. The safety feature of such a machine is especially beneficial for those training alone.

This exercise is also often performed using free weights (Photo 6.2).

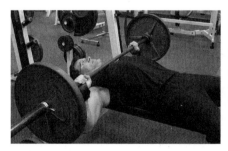 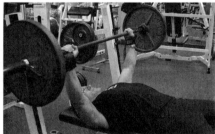

(Photo 6.2) The standard Barbell Bench Press using free weights.

Use a spotter whenever performing the bench press as it is not uncommon for people to misjudge their capabilities and find themselves pinned under a heavy bar that they are unable to return to the support arms.

Flat Dumbbell Press

Starting Position
Sit on the end of a flat bench with both dumbbells resting on your knees. Set your feet approximately shoulder width apart.

To bring the weights into position for your set, hold the weights in position against your knees as you roll backwards on the bench. As you complete this maneuver, your arms should be almost straight up toward the ceiling with the dumbbells held directly above the shoulder joint.

Your hands should be in a palms forward position. Remember, these hand position designations are a general guideline. As we discussed previously, your actual hand position may vary by 10–20 degrees as appropriate for your personal physique.

Movement
1. While being sure to keep your upper arms at right angles to your torso, slowly bend your arms and lower the weights until they are at your chest level.

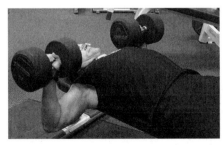

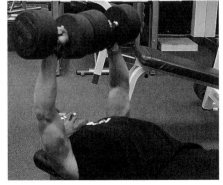

(Photo 6.3) Flat Dumbbell Press

2. Press the weights back, upward along the same arc of travel until your arms are almost straight. Do NOT lock out your elbows in the top position.

3. Repeat for the desired number of repetitions.

Comments

Although proper breathing is probably second nature to you by now, it does not hurt to inject reminders from time to time. With this pressing movement, you should be exhaling as you push the weights upwards and inhaling as you bring them back down.

Seated Chest Press Machine

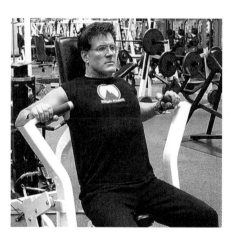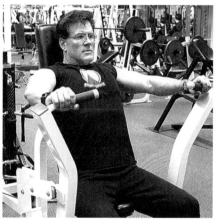

(Photo 6.4) Seated Chest Press Machine

Starting Position

Position the adjustable chair and handles such that your elbows are out to the sides when you bring the bar backwards. In the starting position you should be able to envision a line connecting your hands. This imaginary line would cross your chest at approximately the nipple line. Be sure to keep your shoulders pulled back and your chest out. In order to ensure that you will be using a full range of motion, your hands should

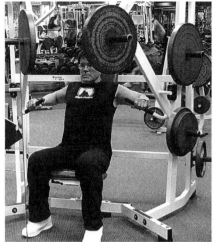 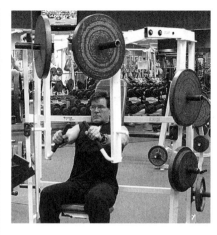

(Photo 6.5) Different companies offer their own versions of the Seated Chest Press Machine.

be far enough back such that if you were holding a physical bar, it would be touching your chest.

Movement

1. Push the weight forward until your arms are just shy of being fully extended. Be sure to keep your shoulders pulled back so that your chest muscles and not your frontal deltoids are doing the work.

2. Slowly return the weights to the starting position. Repeat this motion for the desired number of repetitions.

Comments

As you may have already noticed, the seated chest press machine is almost the same exercise as the basic flat bench barbell press. The seated machine version offers the convenience of sitting in an upright position instead of lying down. Another nice feature of the seated chest press is the simplicity and speed of selecting the amount of weight being lifted with the pin and stack system.

One mistake I see people make all the time when performing this exercise is using an incorrect seating position that places their elbows in a position much lower than their shoulders. Be sure to keep your elbows flared out to the sides as demonstrated in the above photo. This position will help keep the focus on the chest muscles and avoid improper shoulder rotation.

There are several companies who manufacture variations of this machine. Feel free to experiment with each version offered at your gym or fitness facility.

Seated Pec Machine

Starting Position
Adjust the arms of the machine so that they are opposite each other at approximately the 9 o'clock and 3 o'clock positions. Adjust the seat so that in the starting position your elbows and shoulders are at approximately the same height. Grab the handles with your shoulders back and chest forward.

Movement
1. Maintaining a slight bend in your elbows, bring your hands together in front using a motion similar to hugging a tree trunk. You should feel the work being performed by the inner portion of your chest (pectoral) muscles.

2. Slowly return the handles to their starting position on either side of your body. You should maintain resistance on the chest muscles at all times during this movement.

3. Repeat for the desired number of repetitions.

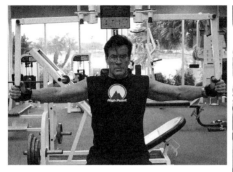
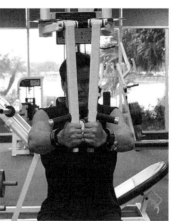

(Photo 6.6) The Seated Pec Machine exercise can be performed using both arms together or only working a single side at a time.

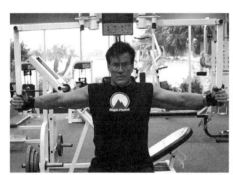
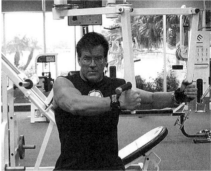

This second variation allows for a wider range of motion across the chest and thus a stronger contraction in the pectoral muscle.

Comments

As with all chest exercises, be sure to prevent your shoulders from shifting forward and causing your chest to cave in. This will take resistance off the chest and place the workload on the frontal deltoids.

If you wish to increase the intensity of this exercise and get even more benefit, you can work one side at a time. When only one arm is being moved, you are not limited to stopping the motion directly in front of your eyes where both hands normally meet. With the single arm motion, you can cross the working hand until it is in the region of the opposite shoulder and thus increase the "squeeze" and tension on the inner pectoral muscle. This variation is in fact my personal preference for getting the most from this movement.

Dumbbell Flyes

Starting Position
Select two appropriately heavy dumbbells and sit at the end of an exercise bench. Raise the weights so they rest on your knees. Roll backwards on the padded bench, simultaneously bringing the dumbbells up to a position on either side of your chest. With your hands in a "palms facing each other" position, bend your elbows 10–20 degrees. Be sure to maintain this bend in your elbows throughout the full movement.

At the starting position, you should now be holding the dumbbells out to the sides of your chest with your upper arms perpendicular to your torso. You should feel a slight amount of stretch in your pectoral muscles.

Movement
1. Maintaining the bend in your elbows, bring the dumbbells upward in an arc until they touch each other.

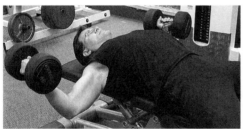

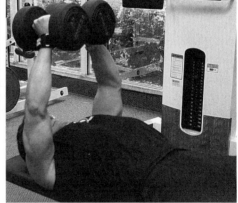

(Photo 6.7) Dumbbell Flyes (flat bench version)

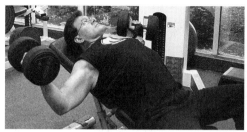
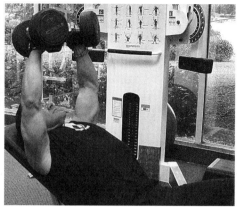

(Photo 6.8) Dumbbell Flyes (incline version)

2. Slowly follow the same arc of motion as you return the weights to the starting position. Be careful not to over stretch or lower the dumbbells too far on the return trip downward.

3. Repeat for the desired number of repetitions.

Comments
Dumbbell flyes can also be performed on an incline bench. Using an incline bench will shift emphasis to the upper section of the chest. For the sake of variety, you are encouraged to alternate between flat and incline flyes every few workouts.

Cable Crossovers

Starting Position
Attach a single grip handle to each of two overhead pulleys. Stand between the pulleys with your feet shoulder width apart. Bend slightly forward at the waist. You will maintain this slight bend during the entire movement.

Your arms at this point should be upwards and back slightly towards the pulley. Your hands should generally be in an 11 o'clock and 1 o'clock position. This hand position is approximately a palms facing position,

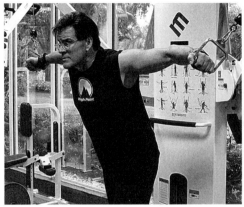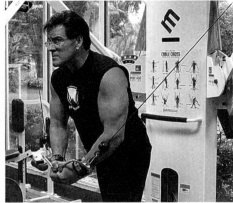

(Photo 6.9) Cable Crossovers

but incorporating the natural angles of biomechanics we discussed earlier (see photo 6.9). Keep your arms slightly bent throughout the entire exercise.

Movement

1. Using your pectoral muscles, pull your arms forward in an arc. The motion should resemble a wide bear hug. Your hands should meet about 6 inches in front of your hips. Let your hands touch.

2. Hold this "squeezed" position for a full second.

3. Slowly return your hands backwards along the same wide arc to the starting position.

4. Repeat for the desired number of repetitions.

Comments

Depending on the length of the cables on the machine at your facility, this movement can be performed either standing or in a kneeling position. Care should be exercised when returning the cables to the starting position. While you want the chest muscles to get a nice stretch and full range of motion, you don't want to allow the hands to go backward too far. Excessive motion of the arms backward could injure the pectorals or shoulder.

SHOULDERS

The combination of exercises below will work the frontal, side, and rear deltoids. Many people neglect to exercise the rear head of the shoulder. This oversight sometimes leads to unbalanced development of the shoulder muscles. Exercising the rear deltoid helps to prevent bad posture and the hunched forward look many people develop in later years.

First Exercise Movement
Machine Shoulder Press
Dumbbell Shoulder Press

Second Exercise Movement
Dumbbell Lateral Raises
Lateral Shoulder Machine

Third Exercise Movement
Rear Deltoid Machine
Bent Over Rear Deltoid Raises

Choose **one** exercise from each of the lists above.

For each exercise, perform 1 warm up set of 20 reps followed by 3 working sets of 12-10-8 reps.

The detailed description and photo demonstration for each exercise are as follows:

Machine Shoulder Press (described in previous chapter)

Dumbbell Shoulder Press (described in previous chapter)

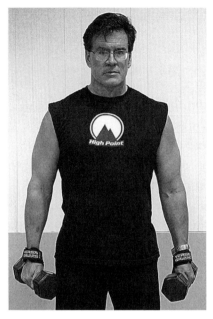

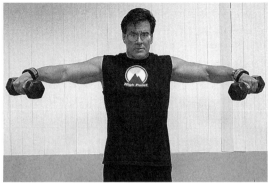

(Photo 6.10) Dumbbell Lateral Raises

Dumbbell Lateral Raises

Starting Position
Grab two light–medium weighted dumbbells and stand with your feet slightly less than shoulder width apart. With your shoulders relaxed and pulled back, bend your arms 10–15 degrees. Relax your wrist so that they drop forward slightly. You should now be in a position that resembles carrying a paint can in each hand.

Movement
1. While maintaining the bend in your elbows, raise your arms upward at each side in a motion similar to a bird flying. Keep your wrist slightly relaxed during the entire movement as though holding two imaginary paint cans.

2. Stop the upward motion when your elbows are at the same height as your shoulders. At this point, your wrists should still be slightly lower than your elbows.

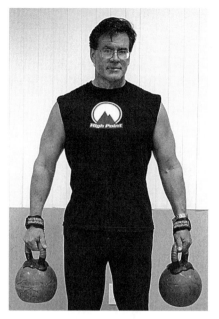

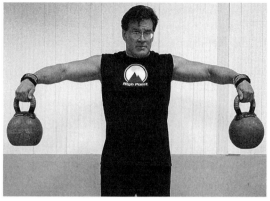

(Photo 6.11) Lateral Raises may also be performed using Kettlebells or Cable Machines.

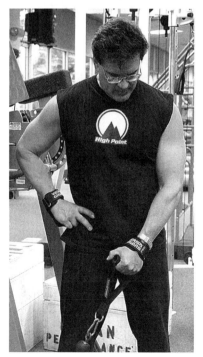

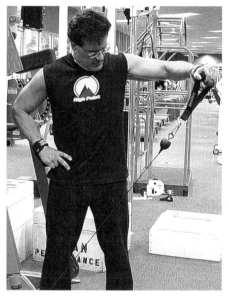

3. Slowly return the weight to the starting position.

4. Repeat this motion for the desired number of repetitions.

Comments

The description and photographs for this exercise may be different than what you have witnessed or been told in the past. There is a good reason for this deviation. Many people complain of outer elbow pain. Commonly called tennis elbow, this inflammation of the lateral epicondyle can make even lifting a carton of milk or shaking hands painful. In some cases, the pain radiates down the forearm and weakens grip strength.

Whenever you lift a weight laterally with a straight wrist and bring the wrist higher than your shoulder, the focal point of strain is shifted to the elbow joint. Such a movement will only aggravate elbow tenderness if it already exists. Using the wrist position and range of motion I described above will take strain off the elbow and keep the focus on the side deltoids.

If your gym offers Kettlebells, you may find these easier to use for this exercise. The Kettlebell naturally places the hands in our desired "carrying paint cans" position.

For variety, lateral raises may also be performed using cable machines. I encourage you to try all these variations.

Lateral Shoulder Machine

Starting Position

Adjust the height of the seat so your shoulders are aligned with the designated pivot points when in a sitting position. Place your forearms under the padded arms and lightly grasp the handles.

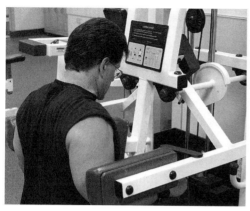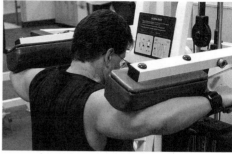

(Photo 6.12)
Lateral Raises Shoulder Machine

Movement

1. Raise your arms outward and upward in a semicircular arc until your elbows are at shoulder level.

2. Slowly return weights downward to the starting position.

Comments

The lateral shoulder machine duplicates the motion of lateral dumbbell raises, but is easier for some people who have difficulty maintaining proper form with the free weight version. Some people with lateral elbow pain find this machine version uncomfortable since the pads rest on the outer forearms.

Rear Deltoid Machine

Starting Position

Move the two arm attachments on the machine to their rearmost position. Face the machine and adjust the seat so that when seated and holding the handles, your hands, elbows, and shoulders are at the same level.

Place your chest firmly against the padded support. Hold the handles while maintaining a 10–15% bend in your elbows. This slight bend should be maintained throughout the entire movement.

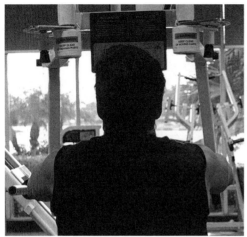

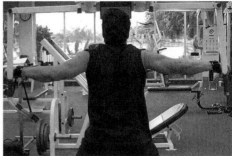

(Photo 6.13)
Rear Deltoid Machine

Movement

1. Using only your rear deltoid strength, pull the arms backwards in an arc. Stop when your hands have moved slightly behind your shoulders. You should feel the muscle contraction in the rear shoulder region.

2. Slowly return your hands along the same arced motion to the starting position.

Comments

Many times the rear deltoid is also performed on the seated pec machine. This piece of equipment is one of many that allows for more than one exercise movement by simply adjusting a few pins and seat positions.

Bent Over Rear Deltoid Raises

Starting Position

Hold two dumbbells while standing with your feet approximately shoulder width apart. Bend forward so that your torso is parallel with the floor. Be sure to maintain a healthy arch in your lower back. Keeping a

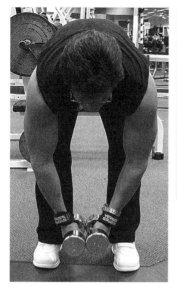
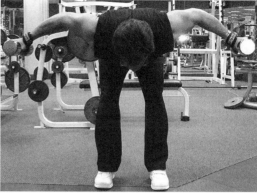

(Photo 6.14)
Bent Over Rear Deltoid Raises

slight bend in your legs will usually aid in maintaining proper position. Allow your arms to hang straight down from the shoulders with your palms facing each other. Bend your elbows 10–15 degrees. The dumbbells should be touching each other at this point.

Movement

1. Using only the strength of your rear deltoids, lift the dumbbells in a semicircular arc directly out to the sides and upwards.

2. Stop when your hands are at shoulder level.

3. Hold this position for a moment, and then slowly return the weights to the starting position.

Comments

Most people will find the previously described machine version of this exercise easier than the free weight movement described here. This rear shoulder movement is very effective, but requires a fair amount of balance and coordination to perform properly.

One common mistake seen in this movement is a tendency to raise the weights to the rear instead of directly out to the sides. This mistake diverts focus away from the rear deltoid and recruits more triceps muscle. As long as you remember to maintain your body and arms in a T-shaped position, you should really feel this exercise concentrated in your rear shoulder muscles.

TRICEPS

The triceps are a smaller muscle group than either the chest or shoulders. Since the arms receive stimulation when exercising these other body parts, we only need to perform 6 working sets for triceps.

First Exercise Movement
Triceps Pulley Pushdowns
Triceps Extension Machine
Triceps Dips Machine

Second Exercise Movement
Overhead Barbell Triceps Extensions
Lying Barbell Triceps Extensions
Triceps Kickbacks

Choose **one** exercise from each of the lists above.

For each exercise, perform 1 warm up set of 20 reps followed by 3 working sets of 12-10-8 reps.

The detailed description and photo demonstration for each exercise are as follows:

Triceps Pulley Pushdowns (described in previous chapter)

Triceps Extension Machine (described in previous chapter)

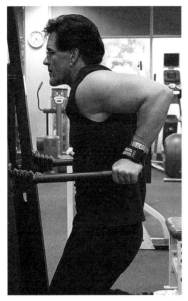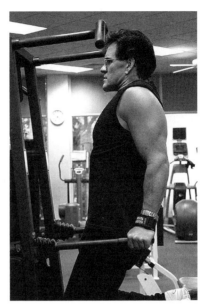

(Photo 6.15) Triceps Dips Machine

Triceps Dips Machine

Starting Position

Select the appropriate counter-weight that will provide suitable resistance.

Depending on the machine being used, adjust either the knee pad or seat so that your upper arms are close to your body and your elbows are directly behind you. Your arms should be fully bent at the elbow with your upper arms parallel to the floor.

Hold you upper body erect with a healthy arch in your spine.

Movement

1. While maintaining your upper torso position, use your triceps strength to straighten your arms until they are just shy of being fully straight.

2. As always, do not lock your elbow joints in the fully extended position. Slowly bend your arms to return to the starting position.

Comments

There are two important things to remember when performing this movement. First, be sure to keep your upper torso straight and perpendicular to the ground. Second, keep your arms close to your body with the elbows behind you. If you allow yourself to lean forward and/or let your arms flare out wide to the sides, the movement becomes more of a pectoral (chest) exercise.

There are two different versions of this machine. On one model, the user lifts their own bodyweight. The weights selected are actually a counter-weight that subtracts from the total resistance. This is helpful since only very strong individuals are able to lift their entire body using only triceps strength for numerous repetitions.

The seated version of this machine is more comfortable for some individuals. On these models, the weight selected is like any other weight resistance machine. The amount you select is the amount you are lifting. Usually a lap belt is featured on these latter versions to keep the user secured in the seat. If your facility offers both versions, you may wish to try both and feel the subtle differences in feel and focus.

Overhead Barbell Triceps Extensions

Starting Position

Place an appropriate amount of weight on the cambered curl bar. Use weight clamps on each end of the bar to secure the plates. Using an overhand grip, rest the bar on your knees while sitting down on a gym seat equipped with a lower back support.

Bring the curl bar up and behind your head with your elbows pointed up towards the ceiling.

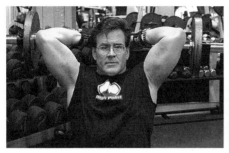

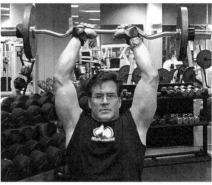

(Photo 6.16) Overhead Barbell Triceps Extensions

Movement

1. Keeping your upper arms motionless and your elbows pointed towards the ceiling, use the strength of your triceps to raise the bar straight over your head.

2. Slowly return the weight back to the starting position while maintaining tension on the back of your arms.

Comments

There are many variations of this exercise. You will see people perform this motion in a standing position, as well as using cables or dumbbells.

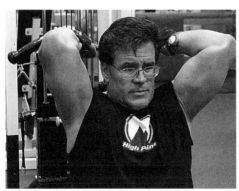

(Photo 6.17) Overhead Triceps Extensions may also be performed sitting in front of a low pulley machine. I personally prefer this cable version.

Training with many people over the years, I have seen that most individuals are better able to maintain proper form when they use some form of supported seated position. The seat allows good lower back support, while the curl bar allows the wrists and forearms to follow a natural range of motion that is easier on the joints.

If your gym has pressing seats with back supports that can easily be moved, you may wish to try this motion sitting with your back to a cable pulley machine. The motion is identical to using the curl bar, but some people are more comfortable with the pulley machines. In this variation, you will adjust the height of the pulley and handle attachment such that when you reach behind you, it is at the appropriate starting position.

Lying Barbell Triceps Extensions

Starting Position
Place an appropriate amount of weight on the cambered curl bar. Use weight clamps on each end of the bar to secure the plates. Using an overhand grip, sit on the end of a flat bench with the barbell resting on your knees. Keep your feet firmly planted on the floor for support.

Lie back on the bench while extending your arms directly upward from your shoulders. At this point, you should be lying flat on the bench with the curl bar held straight up in the air in front of your eyes.

Movement
1. Keeping your upper arms motionless and your elbows pointed towards the ceiling, use the strength of your triceps to lower the bar in a semicircular arc.

2. Stop when the back of your hand lightly touches your upper forehead.

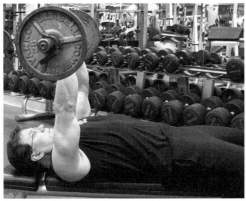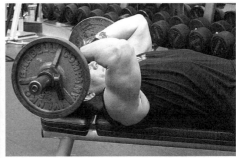

(Photo 6.18)
Lying Barbell Triceps Extension

3. Return the weights to the top position by straightening your arms along the same semicircular arc.

Comments

The cambered curl bar allows the wrists to position and move along a natural range of anatomical motion. You can alternate between the wide and narrow hand positions to shift focus between the three heads of the triceps.

Most exercises for triceps are based on some form of extension. However, the muscles are worked somewhat differently when the pressing motion is performed downwards versus overhead. Once again, variety is highly suggested not only to avoid boredom, but also to provide a well-rounded exercise regimen.

Triceps Kickbacks

Starting Position

Grab a dumbbell in your right hand. Place your left knee and left hand on a flat bench for support. Keep your right foot firmly planted on the floor. Bend until your torso and right upper arm are parallel to the floor. Your elbow should be bent 90 degrees with the forearm perpendicular to the ground.

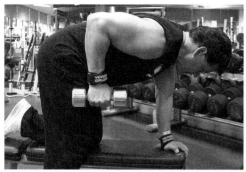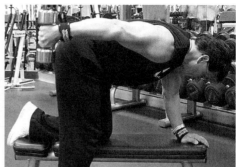

(Photo 6.19) Triceps Kickbacks

Movement

1. Keeping your upper arm close to your body and parallel to the ground throughout the entire movement, use your triceps muscles to straighten your arm out behind you.

2. When your arm is almost perfectly straight, slowly return to the starting position.

3. Once the desired number of repetitions has been performed, mirror and repeat this movement for the other side.

Comments

Because kickbacks are better for toning than developing size and strength, they are a favorite exercise for women. The combination of triceps pulley pushdowns and kickbacks are a popular combination for female trainers.

Men generally tend to prefer the triceps exercises that allow them to push a heavier weight since strong arms have always been a desirable trait for the classic male physique.

For variety, I urge both sexes to include kickbacks every few weeks in their exercise rotation. However, if I were a fly on the wall, I predict I would see the women utilizing this exercise more often than the men.

MIDSECTION

When it comes to working the midsection, you already know what to do. The same combination of exercises you have already been performing will continue to serve you well at this stage.

Crunches
Leg Raises
Lower Back Hyperextensions

Perform 1 set of 20 reps for each exercise

CARDIO

As with the midsection, the half hour of cardiovascular exercise you have been performing until now is still as good as gold.

Treadmill OR Elliptical Machine

Perform 30 minutes in your Target Heart Range.

Remember to incorporate variable intensity and speed during the thirty minute duration.

That's it for day one! Now head home, clean up, and enjoy the rest of your day.

Assuming your schedule allows you to space your workouts with at least one day's rest in between training days, we will meet back here in 48 hours to work your next group of body parts.

Day 2: Quadriceps, Hamstrings, Calves

We have already discussed the importance of strong legs in the previous chapters. All too often with age, people lose independence and mobility. The ability to simply get around, which we took for granted in our youth, becomes so much more valuable to us as we grow older. Broken hips, bad knees, weak ankles, and other ailments are something all of us fear and wish to avoid if possible.

There are two reasons we group all the muscles of the lower body together in our training profile:

• Our upper body is still recovering from the training we first performed earlier this week. More recovery time is needed before revisiting the upper body and training the muscle groups not targeted on day one.

• The quadriceps, hamstrings, and calves work in concert with each other whenever we walk, sit, run, squat, climb stairs, or simply stand.

It makes sense to train these muscles together on the same day in a coordinated fashion since they also function that way in everyday life.

WARM-UP

Prior to beginning weight resistance training for the day, perform the same 5 minute warm up routine you have already been using.

QUADRICEPS

Since the quadriceps is the largest muscle group being worked on this day, they will be exercised first. As always, we want to protect the knees by performing warm up movements first.

Warm Up Movement
Leg Extensions

First Exercise Movement
Angled Leg Press
Seated Leg Press

Second Exercise Movement
Seated Adduction Machine
Seated Abduction Machine

First perform 3 warm up sets of leg extensions as described earlier. For each warm up set, perform 20 repetitions of a light to moderate weight that serves to loosen the knee and surrounding connective tissue while avoiding hard effort or exertion.

Following the warm up movement, choose **one** exercise from each of the lists above.

For the first exercise movement, perform 1 warm up set of 20 reps followed by 6 working sets of 12-12-10-10-8-8 reps.

For the second exercise movement, perform 1 warm up set of 20 reps followed by 3 working sets of 12-10-8 reps.

Note this is a small variation from our usual pattern. The reason for this is the quadriceps muscles respond best to more sets of a powerful compound pressing motion like leg presses.

The detailed description and photo demonstration for each exercise is as follows:

Angled Leg Press (described in previous chapter)

Seated Leg Press (described in previous chapter)

Seated Adduction Machine

Starting Position
Sit in the machine with the adjustable knee pads in the closed middle position. With your feet flat on the pedals, and your knees bent 90 degrees, rest your knees on the outside of each pad. Using the adjusting arm, slowly swing the knee pads outward.

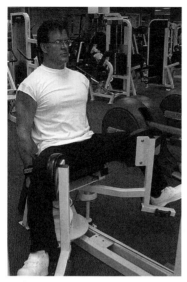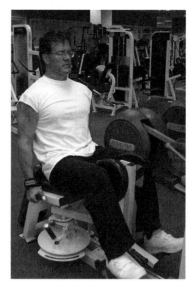

(Photo 6.20) Seated Adduction Machine

Continue to move your legs outwards until you reach the widest stance that gives you a wide range of motion without overextending. Select an appropriate weight using the selector pin.

Movement

1. Using the muscles of your inner thigh, squeeze your legs together until the knee pad support arms touch each other.

2. Hold this position for a moment before slowly moving your legs back outward to the starting position. Be sure to maintain a smooth constant tension on the machine at all times.

Comments

This is an excellent movement for exercising the often neglected inner thigh muscles. Even in people with otherwise good leg conditioning, it is still common to see a lack of muscle tone in the upper inner thigh region between the legs.

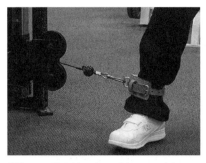 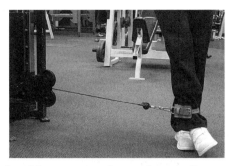

(Photo 6.21) A cable machine and ankle strap can be used to perform this exercise where the specialized equipment is not available.

Before the introduction of specialized weight machines, it was common to see this exercise performed on cable machines utilizing an ankle strap. For gyms not equipped with the pictured machine, the older cable version can still be used (see Photo 6.21).

Historically this exercise was more popular with women, but in recent years men have learned the benefit of this exercise in maintaining balanced leg development.

Seated Abduction Machine

Starting Position
Sit in the machine with the adjustable knee pads opened just wide enough for you to fit your knees in between them. With your feet flat on the pedals, and your knees bent 90 degrees, rest your knees on the inside of each pad. Using the adjusting arm, slowly close the knee pads inward. Select an appropriate weight using the selector pin.

Movement
1. Using the muscles of your outer thighs and hip, move your legs outward until they are as wide as is comfortable for your natural range of motion.

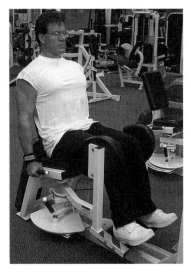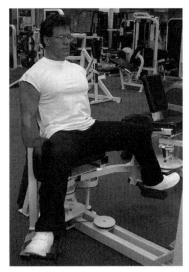

(Photo 6.22) Seated Abduction Machine

2. Hold this position for a moment before slowly moving your legs back inward to the starting position. Be sure to maintain a smooth constant tension on the machine at all times.

Comments

This is an excellent movement for exercising the often neglected outer thigh and hip muscles. As with the adduction movement above, it was common to see this exercise performed on cable machines utilizing an ankle strap in the past. For gyms not equipped with the specialized equipment, you are certainly welcome to use the cable version.

This exercise has also been historically more popular with women, but men now know the benefit of this exercise in maintaining balanced leg development.

As you may have already guessed, it is a good idea to alternate between the adduction and abduction movements every few workouts.

HAMSTRINGS (back of leg)

The hamstrings receive a fair amount of indirect stimulation when the quadriceps muscles are worked with pressing movements. For this reason, you only need to perform 6 working sets for this body part. Since there are only a few exercises available for working the hamstrings, you will see that your options for variety are more limited.

First Exercise Movement
Lying Leg Curl

Second Exercise Movement
Seated Leg Curl
Standing Leg Curl

Choose **one** exercise from each of the lists above.

For each exercise, perform 1 warm up set of 20 reps followed by 3 working sets of 12-10-8 reps.

The detailed description and photo demonstration for each exercise are as follows:

Lying Leg Curl (described in previous chapter)

Seated Leg Curl (described in previous chapter)

Standing Leg Curl

Starting Position
Stand facing the machine while using the supports to stabilize your upper body. Some models feature hand grips while other manufacturers utilize a forearm rest pad to lean on.

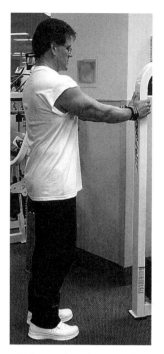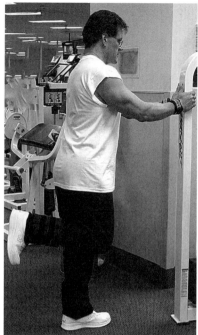

(Photo 6.23) Standing Leg Curl using ankle weights instead of specialized equipment.

Place your right knee against the restraint pad while placing your right heel under the roller bar. Your right leg should now be almost straight with your upper body supported so as to prevent excess movement.

Movement

1. Using only the strength of your hamstrings muscle, curl the roller bar upward so that your leg is bent as far as possible. Be sure to keep your knee in contact with the restraint pad at all times.

2. Slowly return your leg to the starting position.

3. Once the desired number of repetitions has been performed, switch to the opposite side and repeat the process.

Comments

While almost all gym and fitness centers seem to be equipped with both the lying and seated leg curl machines, the standing version is less common.

Before the introduction of specialized weight training equipment, people would perform this exercise using weighted boots. In fact, the fitness facility where the photos for this book were taken did not feature a standing leg curl machine. In the demonstration photo above, I am using ankle weights which are similar in concept to the classic boots I just described.

CALVES

As we have already learned, the calf muscles are worked with a simple up-down motion. After warming up, we incorporate calf raises with a straight leg to focus on the gastrocnemius. Seated calf raises with the leg in a bent position are performed to work the soleus muscles.

Warm Up Movement
Calf Stretch Raises

First Exercise Movement
Calf Machine

Second Exercise Movement
Seated Calf Raises

First perform 2 warm up sets of Calf Stretch Raises as described in the previous chapter. For each warm up set, perform 20 repetitions making sure to use a full and slow range of motion to stretch the Achilles tendon and muscles in preparation for weight-bearing exercises.

Following the warm up movement, choose **one** exercise from each of the lists above.

For each exercise, perform 1 warm up set of 20 reps followed by 3 working sets of 12-12-12 reps.

You are already familiar with all these movements, as they were part of your 30-3 Routine. The only difference now is that instead of alternating between the exercises on different days, you now perform both movements on this leg workout day.

MIDSECTION

Your waist knows this regimen by now:

Crunches
Leg Raises
Lower Back Hyperextensions

Perform 1 set of 20 reps for each exercise

CARDIO

You know what to do. Pick your machine and get moving:

Treadmill OR Elliptical Machine.

Perform 30 minutes in your Target Heart Range. Remember to incorporate variable intensity and speed during the thirty minute duration.

That's day number two completed for this week! Get yourself a high protein drink and head home. I will meet you back in the gym in a day or two for your last training day of the week.

Day 3: Back, Biceps, Trapezius, Forearms

With age, we often see people develop problems with posture as well as a loss of grip strength. On our third and final day of training for the week, we focus on the pulling muscle groups of the body.

WARM-UP

Prior to beginning weight resistance training for the day, perform the same 5 minute warm up routine you have been doing on the previous training days.

BACK

As is always our strategy, we work our largest muscle group first. For today, that will be the back. In order to fully work the back muscles properly, we must perform both rowing motions and pulling (chinning) motions. In your earlier foundation training, you alternated between exercises that would work these different portions of your back. Now that we are using a split routine, you will work your entire back on the same day.

The breakdown of exercise options below will ensure that you always choose a combination of movements that will give you a comprehensive workout.

First Exercise Movement
Seated Pulley Rows
Seated Machine Rows

Second Exercise Movement
Lat Cable Pulldowns
Pull Up - Chinning Machine

Third Exercise Movement
Stiff-Arm Lat Pulldowns
T-Bar Rowing Machine

Choose **one** exercise from each of the lists above.

For each exercise, perform 1 warm up set of 20 reps followed by 3 working sets of 12-10-8 reps.

The detailed description and photo demonstration for each exercise are as follows:

Seated Pulley Rows (described in previous chapter)

Seated Machine Rows (described in previous chapter)

Lat Cable Pulldowns (described in previous chapter)

Pull Up - Chinning Machine

Starting Position
This machine is a weight-assisted piece of equipment. This means that the weight you select on the stack is not equivalent to the amount of weight you are lifting, rather it is the amount of assistance the machine is giving you to help you lift your own bodyweight.

Enter the machine by grabbing the overhead bar with a grip that is 4–8" wider than your shoulders. Rest your knees on the padded weight as-

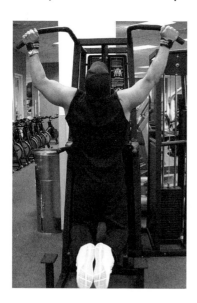
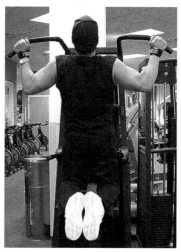

(Photo 6.24) Pull Up – Chinning Machine

sistance mechanism. Keep your upper body straight while maintaining a natural S-bend arch in your lower back.

Movement

1. Focusing on your latissimus dorsi muscles, pull yourself upwards in a chinning motion. Your elbows should flare out to the sides as you perform this movement. Resist the temptation to rotate your elbows to the front of your body, as this will cause your arms to takeover much of the effort.

2. Pull yourself upwards so that your chin is approximately level with your hands.

3. Slowly lower yourself to a point where your arms are almost straight.

4. Repeat for the desired number of repetitions.

Comments

This exercise is excellent since it allows anybody to perform chinning exercises regardless of their upper body strength. The reality is that very few people over age 40 (or any age for that matter) are able to perform multiple repetitions of a full wide-grip chinning motion while lifting their full bodyweight.

You will experience a sense of accomplishment over time as your back and arms strengthen and you find yourself using less assistance from the machine as the months pass.

Stiff-Arm Lat Pulldowns

Attach a long bar handle to the top end of an overhead cable system. Either a straight bar or cambered bar is suitable for this exercise.

Grab the bar with your hands at shoulder width. Bend your arms at the elbows approximately 10 degrees. This bent arm position should be maintained throughout the entire motion as this will prevent stress in the elbow region.

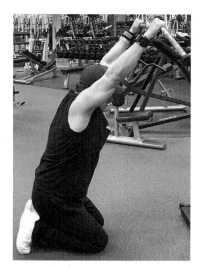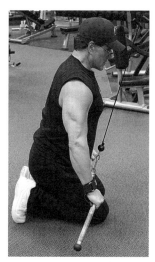

(Photo 6.25) Stiff-Arm Lat Pulldowns

Step back far enough from the machine such that the cable length will allow you to have a full range of resistance from a point where your hands are overhead to the point where they will almost touch your legs in the down position. Stand with your feet shoulder width apart.

Movement

1. While maintaining the 10 degree bend in your elbows, move the bar downward in an arc until it reaches your upper thighs.

2. Slowly return the bar upward along the same arc to the starting position.

3. Repeat for the desired number of repetitions.

Comments

Depending on the design and height of the cable machines at your gym, you may need to perform this exercise from a kneeling position. Taller individuals may also need to perform this exercise from a kneeling position in order to have weighted tension when in the starting position. The goal of this exercise is to maintain tension through the entire range of movement.

T-Bar Rowing Machine

Starting Position

Stand on the machine's platform. With your knees slightly bent, reach forward and grab the handles of the T-bar machine.

Arch your back to maintain the anatomically correct S-bend we have stressed so many times before. Be sure your shoulders are pulled back and not overextending in a forward slouched position.

Movement

1. Without allowing your body to bend forward, pull the bar upward as far as possible.

2. Slowly lower the bar downward toward the starting position. Stop lowering the bar when your arms are just shy of being totally extended. As always, do not lock out your elbow joints.

Comments

I have used the term "T-bar" somewhat loosely in describing this exercise. Over the years, various equipment manufacturers have introduced their own variations of the original "T-bar machine." The version dem-

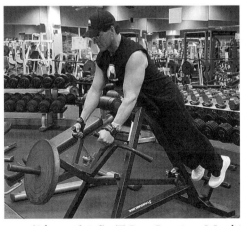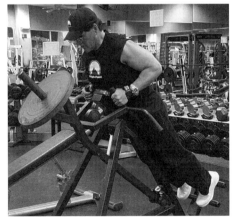

(Photo 6.26) T-Bar Rowing Machine

onstrated in the above photo features a support that braces the upper torso. This support helps prevent strain on the lower back. I find this variation of the basic "T-bar" movement to be a wise choice for we older individuals.

BICEPS

The biceps muscle is often viewed as the symbol of strength. While it may be fun to strike a quick pose and flash a strong arm muscle, the biceps is functionally important for everyday tasks like flipping mattresses, carrying groceries, hauling trash cans to the curb, etc.

Since the biceps muscle is heavily recruited when we train the back, we only need to perform 6 working sets.

First Exercise Movement
Biceps Barbell Curl
Cambered Bar Curl
Dumbbell Curls

Second Exercise Movement
Scott Curls
Concentration Curls
Cable Curls

Choose **one** exercise from each of the lists above.

For each exercise, perform 1 warm up set of 20 reps followed by 3 working sets of 12-10-8 reps.

The detailed description and photo demonstration for each exercise are as follows:

Biceps Barbell Curl (described in previous chapter)

Cambered Bar Curl (described in previous chapter)

Dumbbell Curls (described in previous chapter)

Scott Curls

Starting Position

Place an appropriate amount of weight on either a straight barbell or cambered curl bar. Walk around to the reverse side of a padded preacher bench. Hold the bar with an underhand grip at a distance 1–3 inches wider than your shoulders.

Lean over the preacher bench until the pad is snugly fitted under your armpits. Allow your arms to hang downward toward the floor. Your arms should be almost straight, but not fully extended or locked at the elbows.

Movement

1. Use only the strength of your biceps to curl the weight upward in an arced motion. Raise the weight as high as possible while keeping the back of your arm in contact with the padded bench. For most people this means the forearms will be at close to a 45 degree angle in the topmost position.

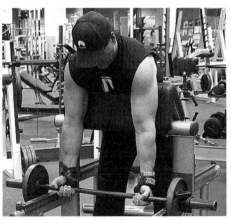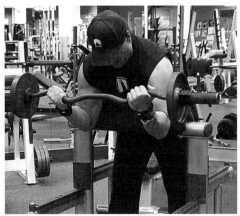

(Photo 6.27) Scott Curls

2. Slowly lower the weight downward to the starting position, being sure to stop just shy of a fully extended hanging position.

Comments

This Scott Curl is a variation of a popular exercise known as the Preacher Bench Curl. The Preacher Bench Curl is performed on this same piece of equipment but using the opposite side of the bench. When performed in this fashion, the upper arm rests in a downward slope on the slanted padded support.

The reason I recommend the Scott Curl over the standard Preacher Bench Curl is a matter of comfort and safety. While an excellent exercise when performed properly, the Preacher Bench Curl causes elbow discomfort for many people. Additionally, extra caution must be used when lowering the weights on the slanted preacher bench to avoid over-extension and biceps tendon injury.

The suggested Scott Curl offers all the training benefits of biceps isolation while avoiding these discomfort and injury concerns.

Concentration Curls

Starting Position

Grab an appropriate dumbbell and sit on the end of a flat bench. Set your feet flat on the floor at a distance 4–6 inches wider than your shoulders.

Bend forward and brace your right triceps against the inside of your right thigh. Rest your left hand on your left knee for support. Allow your right hand and dumbbell to lower to the floor until your arm is almost fully straight.

Movement

1. Use only the strength of your biceps to curl the weight upward in an arc towards your shoulder. Be sure that your arm remains supported by the inside of your thigh throughout the full range of motion. In

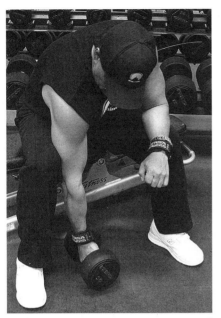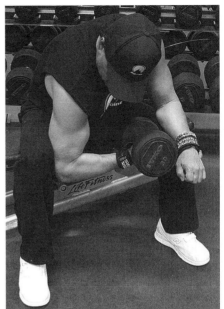

(Photo 6.28) Concentration Curls

fact, if performed properly, your upper arm should remain almost perfectly perpendicular to the floor at all times. Only your forearm should move during this exercise.

2. At the topmost position, tense your flexed biceps slightly.

3. Lower the weight slowly to the starting position.

4. Repeat the motion for your left arm by mirroring this movement.

5. Continue working both arms for the desired number of sets and repetitions.

Comments

Concentration curls can be performed with the palms facing upward OR you can utilize the same pronation and rotation of the wrists we used in standard dumbbell curls to stimulate full function of the biceps muscle.

Cable Curls

Starting Position
Attach either a straight bar or angled bar attachment to the bottom end of a cable pulley machine. Grab the bar at approximately shoulder width using an underhand grip. Step approximately 1–2 feet back from the pulley machine such that you feel tension on the cable when the bar is held in the lowered position.

Stand erect with your feet spaced at shoulder width. Press your upper arms against the sides of your body while envisioning an imaginary pin or rod passing through your body holding your elbows in place on a pivot.

Movement
1. Being careful not to allow your upper body to sway, use your biceps strength to curl the weight upward in an arc towards your upper

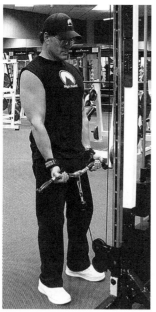 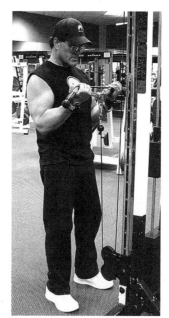

(Photo 6.29) Cable Curls

chest. Do not allow your elbows to leave the sides of your body. In the topmost position, most people will find their hands to be level with, or slightly below, their shoulder level.

2. Slowly return the bar to the starting position, being cautious to avoid total extension of the elbow joint in the bottom position.

3. Repeat for the desired number of repetitions.

Comments

As with most curl movements, the most important thing to keep in mind is to avoid the tendency to lift the weight too high by shifting the elbows forward. When the elbows begin to move in front of the body and weights are lifted towards the chin, the biceps is removed from the motion as the frontal deltoids assume the workload.

Hand position can be varied to place focus on different portions of the biceps muscle. A narrower grip will shift more intensity to the outer sides of the bicep. A wider grip will work the inner side of the biceps to a greater extent. Utilize a variety of hand position widths over time to be sure to fully exercise the biceps muscles.

TRAPEZIUS

Many people don't think of exercising the trapezius muscles at the base of the neck. For those of us in our 40s, 50s, or older, it is wise not to neglect these muscles. In everyday modern life, we don't perform enough lifting motions to keep these muscles properly developed.

Strong trapezius ("traps") are essential for holding the shoulders up, supporting the upper back, and minimizing the tired, slouched appearance we often associate with aging.

While there are a variety of exercises available for exercising the traps, I only recommend the natural motion offered by shrugs.

Exercise Movement
Dumbbell Shrugs

For this exercise, perform 1 warm up set of 20 reps followed by 3 working sets of 12-12-12 reps.

Dumbell Shrugs

Starting Position
Grab two medium heavy dumbbells. With your feet no more than shoulder width apart, stand erect with your shoulders pulled back and the weights hanging at arms length on each side of your body.

Movement
1. Using only the trapezius muscles at the base of your neck, slowly pull your shoulders straight upwards in a shrugging motion similar to that made when saying "I don't know." Be sure all the lifting motion is being performed by the traps and that you are not bending your elbows, or jerking in any way.

2. Slowly lower your shoulders back to their natural position. Do not exaggerate, lower, or slouch your shoulders in any way when returning to the lower starting position.

3. Repeat for the desired number of repetitions.

Comments
Do NOT rotate your shoulders while performing this exercise. Without a doubt, the single biggest mistake people make when performing this motion is to rotate the shoulders instead of shrugging.

Rotating the shoulders will offer minimal benefit to the trapezius, but will greatly increase the probability of rotator cuff or other shoulder injury. I don't know where the bad habit of rotating the shoulders with

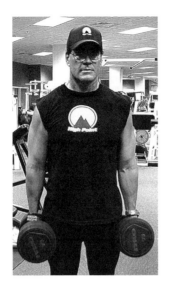 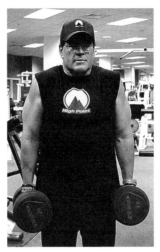

(Photo 6.30) Dumbbell Shrugs

heavy weight got started, but it is a potential injury-inducing movement I see somebody doing every week.

Since the dumbbells remain so close to the body during this movement, most people find it beneficial to remove any large objects like wallets, keys, or phones from their pockets before starting this exercise.

FOREARMS

Although the muscles of the forearms receive a fair amount of stimulation when training the back and biceps, it is still a good idea to dedicate at least one exercise to targeting this all important portion of the lower arm. With age, many people experience a loss of both grip and rotational wrist strength.

The combination of the forearm exercise shown below with the use of a spring hand exerciser at home, will go a long way towards helping you maintain the ability to open jar lids, carry heavy bottles, and use common hand tools.

Exercise Movement
Forearm Cable Curls

For this exercise, perform 1 warm up set of 20 reps followed by 3 working sets of 12-12-12 reps.

Forearm Curls

Starting Position
Place a single handle on the low pulley of a cable machine. Stand erect while stepping slightly off to one side of the low pulley attachment. Your goal is to find the proper position that keeps tension on the forearm when your hand is in the lowered position.

Movement
1. Slowly and firmly curl your wrist forward so that the inner forearm muscles flex and tighten.

2. When you can move no further in this direction, slowly relax the wrist past the original starting point so that you begin pulling your wrist upward and the muscles on the top of your forearm tense and tighten.

3. Continue this back and forth flexion and extension of the wrist for the desired number of repetitions.

4. Repeat for the other forearm.

Comments
There are many different weight exercises commonly used to train the forearms. However, there is a logical reason why I advocate this free standing cable motion over all other movements.

Some other forearm training motions require the forearms to be braced on the knees or supported on the edge of a bench. For many older individuals, these restricted positions create pain and pressure in the elbows as well as stress along the radius and ulna bones of the forearm.

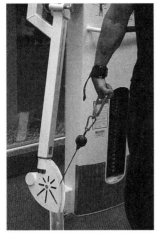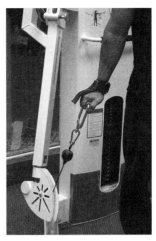

(Photo 6.31) Forearm Cable Curls

The standing cable forearm exercise described here allows the lower arm, wrist, and elbow to coordinate and function in an anatomical position most similar to the way you move in everyday life.

For variety, and to ensure the forearms are exercised from a variety of functional angles, experiment with holding the hands in different positions ranging from palms forward to having the palms facing backward.

MIDSECTION

On this day, we will make a small modification to our usual midsection routine. Having already performed the hyperextension movement for our lower back twice this week, we will substitute an exercise for oblique muscles today. The oblique muscles are located on each side of your midsection.

So get on the floor and knock out the reps.

Crunches
Leg Raises
Side Bends

Perform 1 set of 20 reps for each exercise.

Our newly introduced midsection exercise is performed as follows:

Side Bends

Starting Position
This movement uses the same hyperextension bench that you have been using for your lower back. Position yourself in a sideways position such that your upper body can freely move laterally over the edge of the upper support.

Cross one arm in front of your body (or place that hand behind your head), while the hand of the opposite arm rests on the side of the waist being exercised.

Secure your ankles under the foot support. In the starting position, you should be holding your body straight outwards in the air.

Movement
1. Slowly lower your body laterally until you feel a healthy stretch in your oblique muscle at the side of your waist.

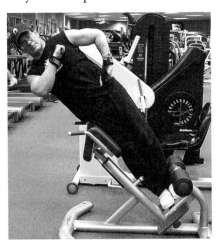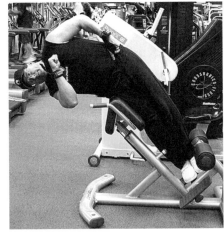

(Photo 6.32) Side bends using hyperextension bench

2. When you reach the bottom, slowly raise your torso back to the starting position. Be sure not to rise too high. You only want to return to the point that your body is straight. Do not reverse flex your waist in the opposite, upward position.

Comments

The reason I stress only raising the torso to a straight position is that most people prefer a tight, slender waist. Working the oblique muscles in the manner I describe helps to tone, stretch, tighten, and smooth them.

When you bend upward too far, you effectively flex, shorten, and "bunch" the oblique muscle. While this certainly works the muscle harder, some people feel this causes the oblique to overdevelop and thicken, causing a wider appearance to the waist.

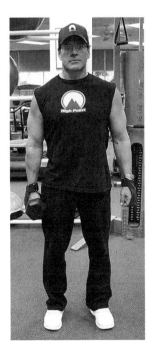
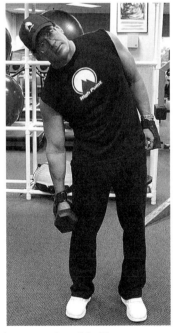

(Photo 6.33) Side bends using dumbbell

A variation of this exercise can be performed with a lightweight dumbbell (see Photo 6.33).

In this version, the dumbbell provides resistance as opposed to the force of gravity on your suspended upper torso. The same rules apply regarding a full lateral stretch downward and only returning upward to a straight standing position.

With either version of this exercise, you should really feel your lateral oblique muscles toning up—especially if you have never performed specialized movements for this region before.

Perform 20 repetitions for each side.

CARDIO

You already know what to do. Pick your machine and get your lungs and heart working.

Treadmill OR Elliptical machine

Perform 30 minutes in your Target Heart Range. Remember to incorporate variable intensity and speed during the thirty minute duration.

Hey, You Did It Again

You have just finished your 3 day split routine for the week. This training regimen, combined with the dietary guidelines covered in the first half of this book, forms the basis of your healthy lifestyle routine.

With the variety of exercises demonstrated, there are scores of different combinations you can create to meet your personal needs and goals for the remainder of your life.

To get an idea how to use this chapter's information to create your own personalized exercise routine, I will now outline a sample program for you to use as a model.

Sample 3 Day Split Routine

On the next three pages, I have detailed a sample workout program for the week.

You may wish to photocopy these routines, take them with you, and use them as a guide until you get familiar with this new split training regimen.

A few comments regarding the sample programs below:

- I have only indicated the Working Sets in the charts below. As we have discussed previously, you should always perform a lightweight warm up set of 20 repetitions whenever you begin a new exercise movement that incorporates weights.

- This sample program demonstrates the correct number of sets and repetitions to be performed per body part, although you will want to substitute exercises frequently for variety.

- Remember to show this program to your personal physician to ensure that it is appropriate for your personal situation.

Different people may have medical conditions or a history of physical injuries that may require some modification to the recommended exercises described in this chapter.

DAY 1

Perform 5-minute Warm Up routine before beginning training.

Perform 1 warm up set of 20 reps when switching to each new weight resistance exercise.

Exercise	Sets	Reps
CHEST		
Incline Dumbbell Press	3	12-10-8
Flat Barbell Press	3	12-10-8
Incline Dumbbell Flyes	3	12-10-8
SHOULDERS		
Machine Shoulder Press	3	12-10-8
Dumbbell Lateral Raises	3	12-10-8
Rear Deltoid Machine	3	12-10-8
TRICEPS		
Triceps Pulley Pushdowns	3	12-10-8
Overhead Barbell Triceps Extensions	3	12-10-8
MIDSECTION		
Crunches	1	20
Leg Raises	1	20
Lower Back Hyperextensions	1	20
CARDIO		
Elliptical Machine (inside Target Heart Range)		30 min

Notes:

DAY 2

Perform 5-minute Warm Up routine before beginning training.

Perform 1 warm up set of 20 reps when switching to each new weight resistance exercise.

Exercise	Sets	Reps
QUADRICEPS		
Leg Extensions (warm up movement)	3	20-20-20
Seated Leg Press	6	12-12-10
		10-8-8
Seated Adduction Machine	3	12-10-8
HAMSTRINGS		
Lying Leg Curl	3	12-10-8
Seated Leg Curl	3	12-10-8
CALVES		
Calf Stretch Raises (warm up movement)	2	20-20
Calf Machine	3	12-12-12
Seated Calf Raises	3	12-12-12
MIDSECTION		
Crunches	1	20
Leg Raises	1	20
Lower Back Hyperextensions	1	20
CARDIO		
Treadmill (inside Target Heart Range)		30 min

Notes:

DAY 3

Perform 5-minute Warm Up routine before beginning training.

Perform 1 warm up set of 20 reps when switching to each new weight resistance exercise.

Exercise	Sets	Reps
BACK		
Seated Pulley Rows	3	12-10-8
Pull Up - Chinning Machine	3	12-10-8
Stiff-Arm Lat Pulldowns	3	12-10-8
BICEPS		
Biceps Barbell Curl	3	12-10-8
Concentration Curls (with wrist rotation)	3	12-10-8
TRAPEZIUS		
Dumbbell Shrugs	3	12-10-8
FOREARMS		
Forearm Cable Curls	3	12-10-8
MIDSECTION		
Crunches	1	20
Leg Raises	1	20
Side Bends (on hyperextension bench)	1	20
CARDIO		
Elliptical Machine (inside Target Heart Range)		30 min

Notes:

Chapter Seven

Training at Home

Alternative Routines for those
Unable to Join a Gym

Unless a person has the money and space to build a fully equipped gym in their own home, I feel strongly that most people will get the best benefit joining a fully equipped fitness facility. Earlier I elaborated on the positive benefits and advantages of training at a gym (wide variety of equipment, social interaction with others, safety of having a professional staff nearby, and more).

However, it is understood that for a variety of reasons, there will be those who are unable to join a nearby fitness center or commercial gym.

In this chapter, I will describe a routine that can be used in the privacy of your own home. For those of you who travel frequently, many of these exercises can be adapted for use on the road.

Basic Equipment Needs

Our assumption in writing this chapter is that you are neither able to join a professional fitness center, or invest a large amount of money to build a private gym inside your own home.

The goal here is to offer a full body exercise routine that requires only a few relatively inexpensive items.

For training at home, you will wish to purchase the following:

Dumbbells
These are available as either individual weights, sets of multiple dumbbells, or a newer version that allows you to adjust the weights through the use of a selection pin.

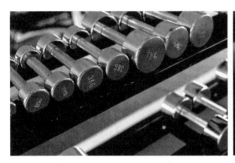 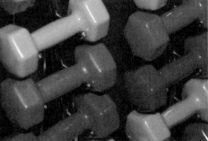

(Photo 7.1) Individual Single Weight Dumbbells

Individual single weight dumbbells are available at a price of approximately $1 per pound. For example, a pair of 15 pound dumbbells will cost around $30.

The advantage of individual single weight dumbbells is their solid construction and comfort. The disadvantage is potential cost and storage space, as you may need to buy several pairs to cover the range of weight required for different exercises.

Vinyl dumbbell sets consisting of individual weights held in place by a locking collar have been around for many years and usually offer the most variety of weight selection for the cost. A 40 pound vinyl dumbbell set can usually be purchased from most retail stores for as low as $20.

The important thing to examine before you buy these is the ruggedness of the locking collar or spring clamps used to hold the weights in posi-

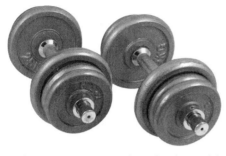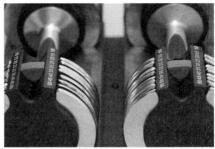

(Photo 7.2) Examples of Adjustable Dumbbells

tion. You want to be sure that the weights will be securely held in place and can not slip off the dumbbell handles when in use.

At an average cost of $250, the new-style adjustable dumbbells may seem more expensive, but they offer the decided advantage of providing the widest variety of weight in a small package. In fact, when one considers the cost and space of buying 18 individual dumbbells at 5 pound intervals to cover the range from 5 to 45 pounds, it quickly becomes evident these newest adjustable weights may be the ultimate option for serious home use.

Hand Exerciser
Spring hand exercisers have been around a long time.

By utilizing different thicknesses of metal coil, the amount of tension can be designed into the exerciser to suit the needs of the user.

Older versions were often sold in a limited number of resistance levels of Light, Medium, or Heavy. Today, these exercisers are available either individually or in sets. A popular set of six hand exercisers ranging from 100 to 350+ pounds of resistance sells for approximately $70.

In actual practice, most people reading this book will only need hand exercisers in the 100–200 pound range of resistance. Once you get into the 250 pound range and higher, you have entered circus strongman territory.

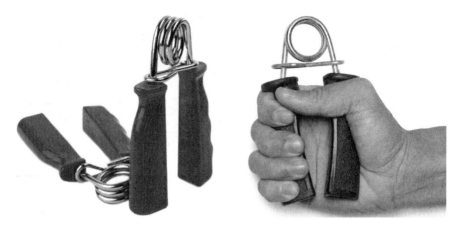

(Photo 7.3) Hand Exerciser

Older individuals with arthritis or those rehabilitating from hand or elbow/forearm tendon injury may wish to find a hand exerciser specifically labeled as light.

Sturdy Wooden Block

I have specified a wooden block here as many people find this easiest to use. It also allows them the portability to perform their exercises anywhere they choose (in the bedroom, living room, on a patio by the pool, etc.).

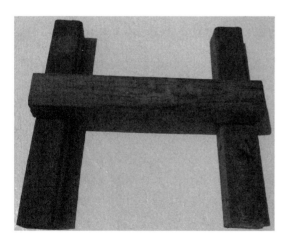

(Photo 7.4) The wooden block should allow for stretching of the heel lower than the toes, while also being stable so as not to move or flip when used. The pictured example was made by bolting together three equal length sections of wood post. Each section measured 24" in length.

Others may have another item around the house that allows for this same purpose. The goal with this item is to provide a way to exercise the calf muscles by stretching the heel lower than the toes. Some people use an old book. This may be acceptable assuming it is sturdy and will not collapse under your weight. Personally, I trust the solid wooden block much more.

Whatever is used, caution must be taken to ensure it is large enough and stable enough not to move or flip when supporting your full bodyweight in motion. Some people use the edge of a step for this purpose, but I hesitate to recommend this. I have known people who have slipped off the step doing this and injured their shins.

A large and stable H-shaped block built by bolting together three equal length sections of wood is a perfect option. This sturdy design gives maximum range of motion for the lowered heel, without raising you higher than necessary off the floor. This style of wooden block is very stable and sturdy.

Ankle Weights

A pair of ankle weights is useful for some of the suggested leg exercises. They will provide the extra resistance you need.

Ankle weights are commonly available in both 5 and 10 pound intervals. You can expect to pay in the range of $15–35 dollars for a pair from most online retailers.

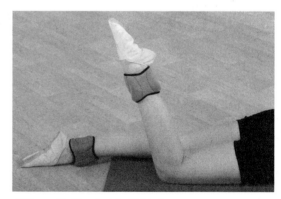

(Photo 7.5) Ankle Weights

Treadmill (Home Style) – Optional

A treadmill is an optional piece of equipment you may wish to consider if you live in a cold climate, work unusual hours, or have problems with self-discipline.

Why do I mention self-discipline? To put it simply, a treadmill helps keep you honest.

Walking is great exercise no matter what pace you use, but as you know from our earlier discussions, the best cardiovascular benefit comes from working 30 minutes inside your Target Heart Rate Zone.

Most people (myself included) find it difficult to maintain an upbeat steady walking stride when they walk around the block, on a nature trail, or around the neighborhood lake. All too often when we walk outside, we start looking at the surroundings, or our mind wanders and we start thinking about other things going on in our lives. The next thing you know, you have started walking much more slowly and are no longer challenging your cardiovascular system.

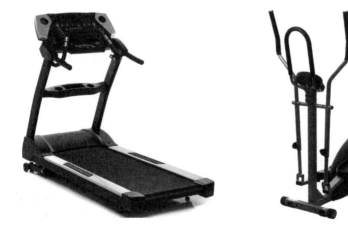

(Photo 7.6) A home treadmill or elliptical is is an optional fitness purchase, but can prove handy in cold climates as well as allow you to perform cardio while watching your favorite TV shows.

An added benefit of having a home treadmill is the ability to watch your favorite TV show while getting your cardiovascular training done for the day. Researchers tell us modern man averages 20–45 hours of TV viewing per week. Most of that time is spent simply sitting or laying on a chair or couch. Watching a single 30 minute sitcom while walking on the treadmill will satisfy that day's requirement for cardiovascular training.

How much can one expect to spend on a simple treadmill for home use? As with most things in life, you get what you pay for. The heavy duty treadmills found in commercial gyms are quite expensive and are probably overkill for the typical home user.

Inexpensive manual treadmills can sell for as low as $150. The limitation and disadvantage of these low end products are usually build quality and the fact that the speed in totally determined by the user. This manual speed limitation introduces the same problem we discussed above with walking outdoors—if your mind wanders, you begin walking more slowly without realizing it.

The preferred style of treadmill is a motorized unit. The motorized unit keeps the treadmill moving at a selected speed, meaning you must maintain your pace to keep up! Expect to pay at least $250 for the least expensive of these models, with more rugged versions starting around $450. Recently manufacturers have also started offering affordable home versions of elliptical machines.

I again wish to point out an indoor treadmill (or elliptical) is not a necessity, but for those really serious about their new fitness regimen, it can certainly be a great investment.

The Home Based Full Body & Cardio Routine

Some readers may already be exercising to some degree while others may not have been physically active in some time.

It is impossible to know the specific and unique physical and medical conditions of every person who may read these words. For that reason, you are urged to show this book to your doctor and discuss the exercises you plan to perform to ensure you have no special conditions that would make the suggested regimen inappropriate for you.

This routine is a full body workout intended to serve as a general conditioning and toning regimen. This routine includes the following features:

- The routine is performed 3 days per week.

- Each major body part is trained with a minimum of 3 sets of a single exercise. Some body parts feature different exercises that you will alternate each training day.

- 30 minutes of cardiovascular training.

You can expect each day of training to take a total of 60–90 minutes including the cardio portion.

You will be working the body in the following order:

- Warm-Up
- Chest
- Shoulders
- Triceps
- Back
- Biceps
- Trapezius
- Forearms
- Quadriceps (front of leg)
- Hamstrings (back of leg)
- Calves
- Midsection
- 30 minutes of Cardio

At the end of the chapter, the entire regimen will be summarized on a single page that you can copy and use as a quick reference guide until you have the program memorized.

WARM-UP

With age, our joints, spine, and connective tissue usually betray the wear and tear of decades long before the muscle tissue itself. For this reason, we want to perform a short warm up routine prior to any strength training exercises.

This series of warm up movements takes less than 5 minutes to perform, and is highly recommended before any strenuous physical exertion.

In fact, if I know I have a full day of yard work ahead of me, I will do this same quick loosening up routine before I grab the wheel barrows, rakes, and shovels.

Shoulder Rotations

Starting Position
Stand with your arms down by your side.

Movement
1. Slowly rotate your arm in a full forward circular motion.

2. As your hand lowers and begins to rotate behind your body, you will need to rotate the wrist. Be sure to rotate the arm through the shoulder's full range of natural motion.

4. Perform the desired number of repetitions. Repeat for the left arm.

5. Repeat the procedure for both arms by rotating the arms in the reverse direction.

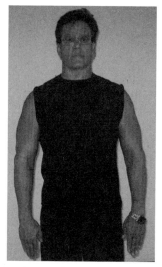 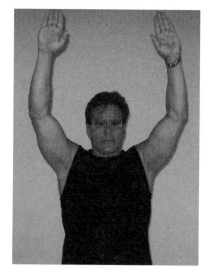

(Photo 7.7) Shoulder rotations (sometimes called windmills) should be performed in a slow, full range of motion. No wild, fast swinging.

Comments

Slow rotation is the important thing to remember with this warm up movement. The focus here is to ensure the shoulder joint and rotator cuffs are flexible and ready for subsequent exercises that require exertion. Do not spin the arms rapidly as you may have done when you were a young child pretending to be an airplane propeller.

Some people prefer to rotate both arms at the same time. Either option is acceptable.

Arm & Elbow Stretches

Starting Position

Stand with your arms and hands positioned as shown in the photo above. The position is similar to how your hands would be held if supporting a heavy tray close to the front of your body. You should have your wrists bent backwards as far as comfortable such that you feel a mild stretch in the wrists and forearms.

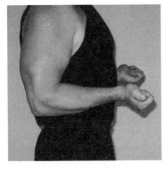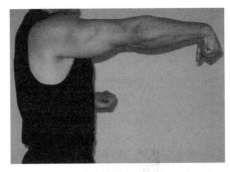

(Photo 7.8) The benefit of this warm up movement exists in the subtle details regarding elbow and wrist motion.

Movement

1. Slowly extend your right arm forward as though you are throwing a punch in slow motion.

2. As your hand moves forward, rotate your wrist so that when you reach full extension, your fist is in a palm downward position.

3. Hold this extended position as you tilt your wrist forward and down toward the floor. You should feel a nice stretch along the top of your forearm extending all the way back to your outer elbow region.

4. Reverse the motion, bringing your arm back to the starting position. You should also rotate your wrists so that by the time your arms are withdrawn, your hands are again in the starting position.

Comments

This is a stretching and warm up exercise that is a bit difficult to accurately describe in a book. Some people may emulate the general motion, but fail to feel the desired stretching in the wrists, elbows, and forearms. The key to getting benefit from this motion is to ensure the wrists are flexed as far as possible until you can feel the gentle stretching extend all the way from the wrists to the elbows.

This motion is similar to a common therapy exercise for people suffering from elbow tendonitis. The benefit to us is that this motion prepares the elbows and wrists for weight-bearing exercises such as pushups, triceps dips, and other movements.

Wrist Rotations

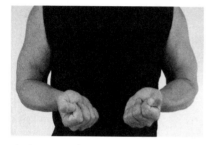
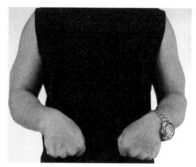

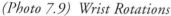
(Photo 7.9) Wrist Rotations

Starting Position
Stand with your elbows bent at a 90 degree angle and your hands in front of your body.

Movement
1. This movement is very simple. Just rotate both wrists for 10–12 repetitions. Most people find it easier to rotate the wrists in opposite directions from each other, such that they are rotating like mirror images of each other.

2. Repeat in the opposite directions.

Comments
This is a very simple motion, but it can be very beneficial to prevent injury. With age, some people complain that their wrists and ankles "get hung up" or otherwise click and pop when working under a load. This gentle warm up motion performed immediately before hard work tends to loosen the wrists and prevent them from experiencing this problem.

Lower Back Stretch

Starting Position
Stand in front of a chair or similar support. Hold the top of the chair (or support) with both hands. Step backwards approximately 3 feet until your arms are straight and you are bending forward slightly.

Movement
1. To stretch the right half of your lower back, drop your left knee slightly while also bending your left arm. This will allow your body to lean to the left and slightly forward (you might think of your head as pointing at the 10–11 o'clock position).

2. As your body leans to the left, your left leg will begin to support more of your bodyweight. You should feel a gentle stretch in the lower back of your right side. When you are in the proper stretched position, your right foot should be slightly forward and resting on the heel. At this point, your right foot will be supporting very little of your bodyweight.

3. Focus on the gentle stretch in your lower back's right side.

4. Repeat this gentle stretching motion 2–3 times before mirror imaging the motion for your left side.

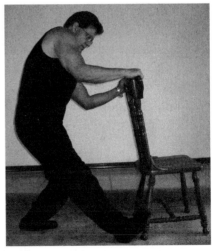

Comments
This is another stretching motion that is easier to demonstrate in a video or in person as compared to a book description. Even the picture above might make it a little diffi-

(Photo 7.10)
Lower Back Stretch Movement

cult to understand the motion, but once you find the right position, you will know it.

Friends of mine with lower back problems or occasional sciatic twinges tell me this helps them loosen up their back before a day of hard work or other physical activity.

Leg and Knee Stretch

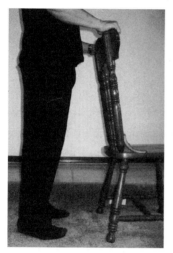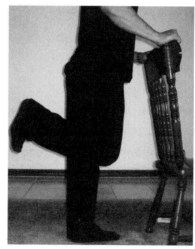

(Photo 7.11) Leg and Knee Stretch

Starting Position
Stand in front of the same chair or support used in the previous movement. Hold the top of the chair (or support) with both hands for stability.

Movement
1. Using the chair back to maintain your balance, slowly bend your right leg up behind you as far as possible. Imagine you are trying to touch your heel to your buttocks.

2. Slowly return your leg to the lower position.

3. In the lower position, tense your frontal thigh muscle while keeping your foot off the floor.

4. Repeat 6–10 repetitions. Do not allow your right foot to return to the floor until you are finished stretching this side.

5. Repeat for the left leg.

Comments
This simple motion limbers up the knees, hamstrings, and frontal thigh for later exercises.

Ankle Rotations

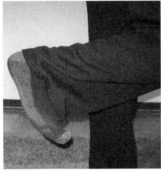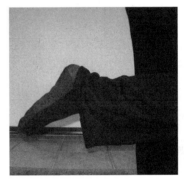

(Photo 7.12) Ankle Rotations

Starting Position
Stand in front of the same chair or support used in the previous two movements. Hold the top of the chair (or support) with both hands for stability.

Movement
1. Lift your right foot slightly off the floor.

2. Rotate your ankle 10 times in a clockwise motion.

3. Repeat the rotation in a counterclockwise direction.

4. Repeat for the left ankle.

Comments

A very simple warm up motion that helps prevent unexpected twisting or collapse of the ankle when walking, running, or doing exercises.

Calf and Achilles Tendon Stretch

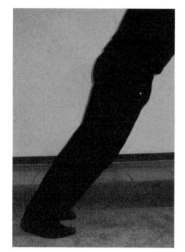 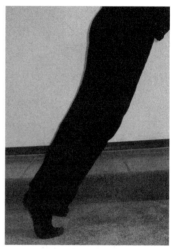

(Photo 7.13) Calf and Achilles Tendon Stretch

Starting Position

Stand with your feet approximately shoulder width apart. Place your hands on a wall for support. Step backwards approximately 3 feet from the wall so that you are leaning forward into the wall. Keep your feet flat on the floor. At this point you should feel a slight stretch to the back of your calves.

Movement

1. Slowly rise up on the balls of your feet while using the wall for support and balance.

2. Slowly lower your heels back to the floor allowing the Achilles tendon, gastrocnemius, and soleus muscles of the lower leg (calves) to stretch.

3. Repeat 10 repetitions or until you no longer feel any tightness in your lower legs.

Comments

With age, it is more important to keep the calves and Achilles tendon flexible to prevent tears or rupture. In Chapter 5, where I first introduced these warm up exercises, I related a real life story regarding muscle tears of the calf. Even if you have no intention of joining a gym or performing the 30-3 or 3 Day Split routines, you may still wish to go back and read that story.

The point is this. At 40 years old and older, we are not the same indestructible creatures we were in our teens.

Do not skip the 3–5 minutes it takes to warm up and stretch your muscles and joints before taking on physical exertion. Warming up is a small, but well spent, expenditure of time.

Now you are primed and ready to begin the exercises.

CHEST

For the chest, we will be performing the classic push up.

Push Ups

Starting Position
Lie facedown on the floor with your hands slightly wider than shoulder width. Flare your elbows out to your sides.

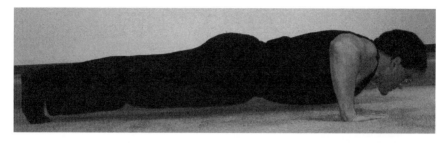

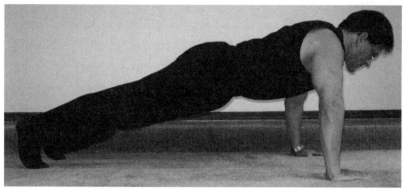

(Photo 7.14) Classic Pushup

Movement

1. Holding your torso firm and straight, push yourself up off the floor until your arms are almost straight. At the top position, your forearms should be perpendicular to the floor.

2. Slowly lower yourself back downwards until your face is only 2 inches from the floor.

3. Perform 3 sets of 10–12 repetitions.

Comments

This exercise is no doubt already familiar to 99.99% of you. It's a classic movement, and still serves as a great equipment-free alternative to bench presses at the gym.

Some individuals may need to perform pushups from their knees instead of their toes until they develop sufficient upper body strength to perform the classic pushup.

If you desire, you can change the portion of the chest, which is targeted by changing the angle at which you perform the movement. If you elevate your upper body higher than your feet, as would be the case when performing pushups on two chairs, the lower chest is worked harder. If you raise your feet higher than your head when performing pushups, you will work the upper chest and frontal deltoids more directly.

SHOULDERS

For the shoulders, you will alternate between two different exercises each time you train. For example, if the first day of the week you perform the dumbbell presses, the next day you work out you will do the lateral raises, etc.

Dumbbell Shoulder Press

Starting Position

Grasp two dumbbells while sitting on a chair that ideally features a support for the lower back. Let the dumbbells rest on your knees as you sit down.

Bring the dumbbells up to a starting position where each weight is held on either side of the head at approximately ear level. Your hands should be in a palms forward position.

Movement

1. Using your shoulder strength, press the dumbbells upward until your elbows are just short of being locked out straight.

2. Slowly lower the weights back to the starting position with hands at approximately ear level.

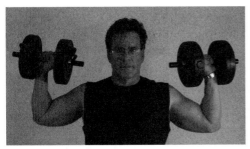

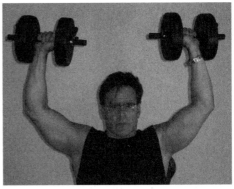

(Photo 7.15) Dumbbell Press for Shoulders

Perform 1 warm up set of 20 reps with a light weight.

Perform 3 working sets of 12-10-8 repetitions.

Comments

This exercise calls for a "palms forward" position. Anatomically each individual may exhibit a few degrees of rotation away from a strict palms forward position. At the risk of sounding repetitive, we must always pay attention to our individual body's joint angles and range of motion. In real life, and especially after 40, 50, 60 or more years of wear and tear, it is natural for us to have a range of motion that varies slightly from a perfect textbook description.

You will notice in the accompanying photograph demonstrating this exercise (Photo 7.15), the hands are essentially in a palms forward position although a slight angle can be detected.

Dumbbell Lateral Raises

Starting Position

Grab two light–medium weighted dumbbells and stand with your feet slightly less than shoulder width apart. With your shoulders relaxed and pulled back, bend your arms 10–15 degrees. Relax your wrist so that

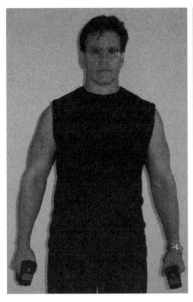
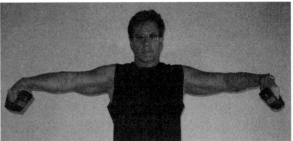

(Photo 7.16) Dumbbell Lateral Raises

they drop forward slightly. You should now be in a position that resembles carrying a paint can in each hand.

Movement

1. While maintaining the bend in your elbows, raise your arms upward at each side in a motion similar to a bird flying. Keep your wrist slightly relaxed during the entire movement as though holding two imaginary paint cans.

2. Stop the upward motion when your elbows are at the same height as your shoulders. At this point, your wrists should still be slightly lower than your elbows.

3. Slowly return the weight to the starting position. Repeat this motion for the desired number of repetitions.

Perform 1 warm up set of 20 reps with a light weight.

Perform 3 working sets of 12-10-8 repetitions.

Comments

The description and photographs for this exercise may be different than what you have witnessed or been told in the past. There is a good reason for this deviation.

Many people complain of outer elbow pain. Commonly called tennis elbow, this inflammation of the lateral epicondyle can make even lifting a carton of milk or shaking hands painful. In some cases, the pain radiates down the forearm and weakens grip strength.

Whenever you lift a weight laterally with a straight wrist and bring the wrist higher than your shoulder, the focal point of strain is shifted to the elbow joint. Such a movement will only aggravate elbow tenderness if it already exists. Using the wrist position and range of motion I described above will take strain off the elbow and keep the focus on the side deltoids.

If you own Kettlebells, you may find these easier to use for this exercise. The Kettlebell naturally places the hands in our desired "carrying paint cans" position.

TRICEPS

For the triceps, you will alternate between two different exercises each time you train. For example, if the first day of the week you perform chair dips, the next day you work out you will do the dumbbell triceps extensions, etc.

Chair Dips

Starting Position
Sit on the edge of a stable and sturdy chair. With your upper arms close to your body, and your elbows pointed straight behind you, grip the edges of the chair on either side of your buttocks.

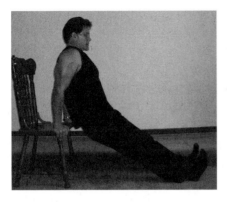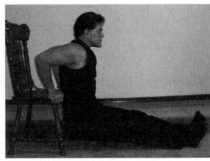

(Photo 7.17) Chair Dips

Rest your heels on the floor with your legs straight in front of you.

Movement

1. Using only the strength of your triceps, lift your body off the chair. Bend your knees slightly so that your upper torso is able to clear the front of the chair.

2. Lower your body towards the floor by slowly bending your elbows. Only lower your body to the point where your elbows are bent approximately 90 degrees and your upper arm is parallel to the floor.

3. Slowly straighten your arms to return to the top position.

Perform 3 sets of 8–12 repetitions.

Comments

DO NOT try to go too low with this exercise. Pay careful attention to the photo and movement description above.

Lowering your body too much can cause excessive rotation and potential injury to the shoulder. Chair dips are an excellent exercise that provides an intense stimulus to all the muscles on the back of the arm, but care must be taken to perform the movement safely.

Focus on keeping your upper arms close to the torso with the elbows pointed straight out behind you. Flaring the elbows or failing to keep the hands slightly posterior to the suspended buttocks will shift focus away from the triceps toward the chest.

Overhead Dumbbell Triceps Extensions

Starting Position

Grab a set of matching dumbbells. Sit on a solid, stable chair. The ideal chair will also offer back support. Rest the weights on your knees.

When you are ready to begin the exercise, bring the dumbbells up and behind your head with your elbows pointed up towards the ceiling.

Movement

1. Keeping your upper arms motionless and your elbows pointed towards the ceiling, use the strength of your triceps to raise the dumbbells straight over your head.

2. Slowly return the weight back to the starting position while maintaining tension on the back of your arms.

(Photo 7.18) Overhead Dumbbell Triceps Extensions

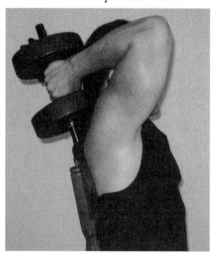
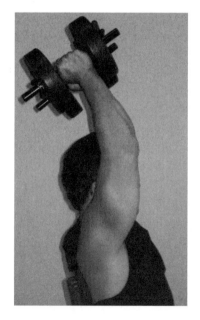

Perform 1 warm up set of 20 reps with a light weight.

Perform 3 working sets of 12-10-8 repetitions.

Comments

This exercise can also be performed in a standing position. If you have a sturdy chair with a good back support available, I recommend using it over the standing option. Training with many people over the years, I have seen that most individuals are better able to maintain proper form when they use the supported seated position I describe above.

Each arm can also be exercised individually in case a matching pair of dumbbells is not available.

BACK

The back is a major body part that is easier to train in a well-equipped gym than at home. However, the one-arm dumbbell row is very effective and will satisfy the needs of most people unable to train at a fully equipped fitness facility.

One-Arm Dumbbell Rows

Starting Position

Place a dumbbell on the floor next to a stable chair. Grab the weight in your right hand and place your left hand on the chair for support and balance. Brace your upper body into position with your torso held parallel to the floor.

Movement

1. Keeping your elbow pointed behind you, slowly pull the dumbbell upward in a motion similar to rowing a boat. Lift the weight as high as possible while maintaining the proper parallel position of the upper body relative to the floor.

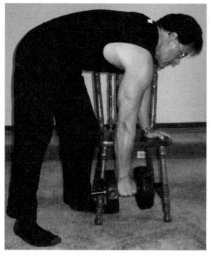
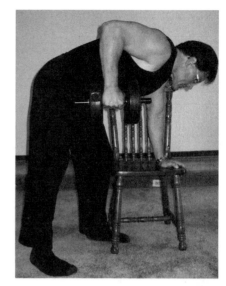

(Photo 7.19)
One-Arm Dumbbell Rows

2. Slowly return the weight to the lowered position.

3. Once the desired number of repetitions has been performed, mirror and repeat this movement for the other side.

Perform 1 lightweight warm up set of 20 reps for each side.

Perform 3 working sets of 12-10-8 repetitions for each side.

Comments

As has been stressed previously, be sure to maintain a natural arch in your lower back. Do not bow or curve the back during this or any other weight-bearing exercise.

Improper bowing or forward curving of the back under a weighted load is one of the most common causes of lower back injuries in our society today.

BICEPS

The good old biceps curl using dumbbells is a great at home exercise for strengthening everybody's favorite arm muscle.

Dumbbell Curls

Starting Position

Grab two appropriately weighted dumbbells and stand erect with your feet positioned at a natural standing width, with your arms hanging down and holding a dumbbell at each side. Hold the dumbbells in a palms upward position.

Press your upper arms against the sides of your body and keep them in this position throughout the full motion.

Movement

1. Without swaying your upper body, use only your biceps strength to curl your right arm upward in an arc. Lift the weight as high as possible without removing your elbow from its position on the side of your torso.

2. As you lower the right dumbbell to its starting position, simultaneously begin lifting the left dumbbell to the raised position.

3. Continue performing this seesaw motion until you have performed the desired number of repetitions for each arm.

Perform 1 warm up set of 20 reps with a light weight.

Perform 3 working sets of 12-10-8 repetitions.

Comments

It is often helpful to hold the dumbbell closer to the end of the bar near your body in order to clear your hips while performing the exercise.

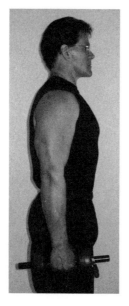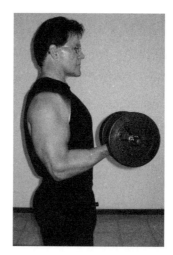

(Photo 7.20) Dumbbell Curls

It is useful to envision an imaginary rod going through your body and holding the elbows in position on either side of your body. There is a natural tendency to try to lift the weights too high (near the chin). This habit causes the elbows to move forward. Once the elbows move forward in front of the body, focus is shifted from the biceps to the frontal deltoids.

Dumbbell curls lend themselves to a wide range of variations. They can be performed in either a standing or sitting position. You can also rotate the wrist midway through the motion to increase intensity on the flexed biceps muscle. Rotating the wrist while lifting offers the added benefit of exercising the biceps through both its normal functions of hand rotation and flexing the arm.

TRAPEZIUS

Strong trapezius muscles are essential for holding up the shoulders, supporting the upper back, and minimizing the slouched appearance we often associate with aging.

Dumbbell Shrugs

Starting Position
Grab two medium–heavy dumbbells. With your feet no more than shoulder width apart, stand erect with your shoulders pulled back and the weights hanging at arms length on each side of your body.

Movement
1. Using only the trapezius muscles at the base of your neck, slowly pull your shoulders straight upwards in a shrugging motion similar to that made when saying "I don't know." Be sure all the lifting motion is being performed by the traps and you are not bending your elbows or jerking in any way.

2. Slowly lower your shoulders back to their natural position. Do not exaggerate, lower, or slouch your shoulders in any way when returning to the lower starting position.

3. Repeat for the desired number of repetitions.

Perform 1 warm up set of 20 reps with a light weight.

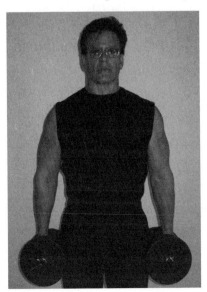
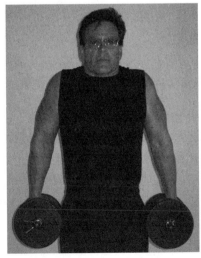

(Photo 7.21) Dumbbell Shrugs

Perform 3 working sets of 12-10-8 repetitions.

Comments

Do NOT rotate your shoulders while performing this exercise. Without a doubt, the single biggest mistake people make when performing this motion is to rotate the shoulders instead of shrugging.

Rotating the shoulders will offer minimal benefit to the trapezius, but will greatly increase the probability of rotator cuff or other shoulder injury. I don't know where the bad habit of rotating the shoulders with heavy weight got started, but it is a technique flaw I see every week.

Since the dumbbells remain so close to the body during this movement, most people find it beneficial to remove any large objects like wallets, keys, or phones from their pockets before starting this exercise.

FOREARMS

With age, many people experience a loss of both grip and rotational wrist strength. The combination of the forearm exercise shown below with the use of a spring hand exerciser will help you maintain the ability to open jars, carry heavy containers, and use everyday hand tools.

I suggest you perform both of these exercises on your training day.

Forearm Dumbbell Curls

Starting Position
Grab a dumbbell in each hand. Stand erect while holding the weights on each side of your body.

Movement
1. Slowly and firmly curl your wrists forward so that the inner forearm muscles flex and tighten.

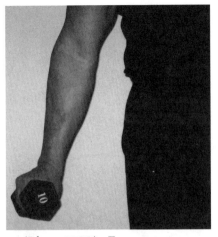
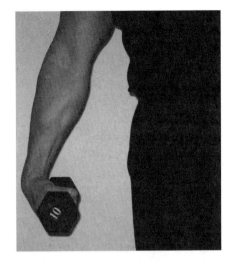

(Photo 7.22) Forearm Dumbbell Curls

2. When you can move no farther in this direction, slowly relax the wrist past the original starting point so that you begin pulling your wrist upward and the muscles on the top of your forearm tense and tighten.

3. Continue this back and forth flexion and extension of the wrist for the desired number of repetitions.

Perform 3 working sets of 12-10-8 repetitions for each forearm.

Comments

Some other forearm training motions you will see described require the forearms to be braced on the knees or supported on the edge of a bench. For many older individuals, these restricted positions create pain and pressure in the elbows as well as stress along the radius and ulna bones of the forearm.

The suspended dumbbell exercise described here allows the lower arm, wrist, and elbow to coordinate and function in an anatomical position most similar to the way you move in everyday life.

For variety, and to ensure that the forearms are exercised from a variety of functional angles, experiment with holding the hands in different positions ranging from palms forward to having the palms facing backward.

Spring Hand Exercisers

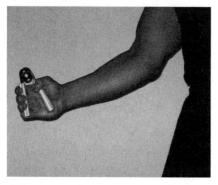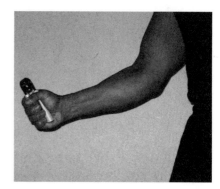

(Photo 7.23) Spring Hand Exercisers

Starting Position
Firmly grab a spring hand exerciser of appropriate tension for your hand strength.

Movement
1. Firmly squeeze the handles as far as possible.

2. Release and repeat.

Perform 3 working sets of 10-10-10 repetitions for each hand.

Comments
Faithful use of spring hand exercisers is very effective at maintaining and even building grip strength as we age.

QUADRICEPS (front of leg)

With age, people really value their independence and mobility. The ability to "get around" that we took for granted in our youth becomes a more valuable gift to us as we grow older.

The frontal leg muscles are vital for everyday activities such as getting up from a chair, climbing stairs, and even walking. The exercises for the quadriceps work these muscles in a manner most similar to their everyday function.

Deep Knee Bends

Starting Position
Stand up straight with your feet positioned approximately shoulder width apart. Allow your toes to angle slightly outwards.

Cross your arms in front of your body and look straight ahead.

Movement
1. While keeping the back properly aligned and straight, lower your body into a deep squat using only the strength of your leg muscles. Be certain NOT to bend at the waist or bow your back forward. All downward motion should come from bending the knees and minor rotation at the hips. Your upper body should remain erect with your head looking straight forward during the entire movement.

Perform 3 sets of 10 to 12 repetitions.

Comments
When explorers visit primitive tribes around the world, they often observe older members of these civilizations still able to squat deeply while working in the fields or collecting water from a river's edge. In our Western civilization, many people acquire the habit of keeping the legs straight and bending over at the waist to pick up items from the floor.

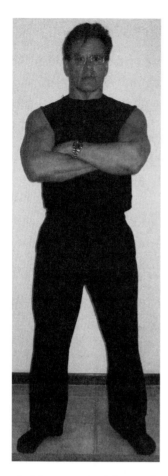

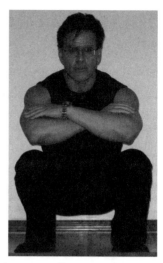

(Photo 7.24) Deep Knee Bends improve flexibility, balance, coordination, and strength in your leg muscles.

It is probably no coincidence that lower back problems are also more prevalent in the civilized world than in primitive regions.

Although no additional weight is called for in this exercise, many readers will find it mildly challenging at first, because most people don't routinely lower their bodies by utilizing a natural squatting motion. The previously mentioned waist bending and back bowing motion is more commonly used in our Western world.

Performing these deep knees bends as described will improve flexibility, balance, coordination, and strength in your leg muscles.

Dumbbell Squats

Starting Position

Grab a dumbbell in each hand. Hold the dumbbells at arm's length on each side of your hips. Stand directly in front of a chair with your legs approximately shoulder width apart. Allow your knees and toes to point slightly outwards. Ensure that the chair selected is an appropriate height that allows your knees to bend 90 degrees when in a sitting position.

Movement

1. Hold your upper torso erect with a natural anatomical arch in your lower back.

2. Slowly lower yourself by bending your legs until your buttocks just barely touch the seat of the chair. Do not sit down or rest. In this exercise the chair is not intended to be used as support. The chair is only to be used as a guide to ensure you consistently squat to a proper depth.

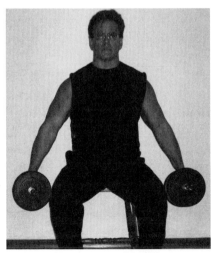

(Photo 7.25) Dumbbell Squats

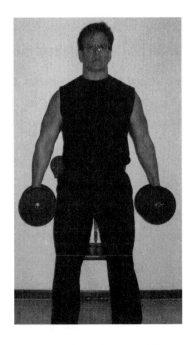

3. Reverse the movement by straightening your legs and returning to the original standing position.

Perform 1 warm up set of 20 reps with little or no weight.

Perform 3 working sets of 10 to 12 repetitions.

Comments

The exercise is essentially nothing more than sitting and rising from a chair with added resistance. The addition of weights helps both strength and balance development.

Optionally, this movement can be made more effective by avoiding the use of a chair, and instead squatting to a deeper position.

Those individuals with a history of knee or lower back problems would be wise to discuss this advanced alternative with their doctor.

The squatting motion performed to a parallel position as described above will be suitable for most home trainers. This is especially true for those well past the age of 50.

HAMSTRINGS (back of leg)

Though sometimes neglected, it is important to exercise the hamstring muscles on the back of the leg. Balanced muscle strength development in the body is important for proper posture and also reducing the chance of injury.

We all know people who have strained or "pulled" a hamstring muscle. This exercise will help improve both flexibility and strength in the back of the leg.

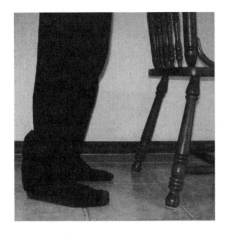
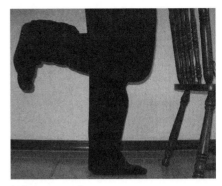

(Photo 7.26)
Standing Leg Curl

Standing Leg Curl

Starting Position
Attach an appropriate sized ankle weight to each leg. Ensure the closure strap is sufficiently snug to prevent the weights from sliding on the lower leg. Stand facing the backside of a chair, using the backrest for balance and support.

Movement
1. Using only the strength of your leg biceps muscle, curl your lower right leg upwards. Bend your leg as fully as possible. Then slowly return to the starting position.

Perform 3 working sets of 10 to 12 repetitions for each leg.

Comments
Many years ago it was common to see this exercise performed using iron boots. These were a special form of shoe upon which weight plates could be attached to add resistance. Today, the ankle weights suggested here are easier to find and more comfortable for most people.

CALVES

The calf muscles are best stimulated with a simple up and down motion using a weighted resistance greater than your bodyweight alone.

One-Legged Standing Calf Raises

Starting Position

For this exercise you will require a dumbbell, the wooden block, and a chair to be used for balance.

Hold your dumbbell in your right hand. Place your right foot on the wooden block so that you will be supporting your weight on the ball of the foot. Balance yourself by placing your left hand on the center of the chair's backrest.

Bend your left leg enough to ensure it will be out of the way during the movement, but is close enough to the ground in the event you lose balance and need to stabilize yourself.

Keeping your right leg straight, allow the weight of your body and additional held weight to push your heel lower than the level of your toes.

Movement

1. While keeping your right leg straight, use the strength of the calf muscle to rise up as high as possible on the ball of your right foot.

2. Slowly return to the lower stretched position. Do not lower too rapidly or bounce.

3. The left calf is trained by performing the mirror image of this description.

Perform 3 working sets of 15 to 20 repetitions for each leg.

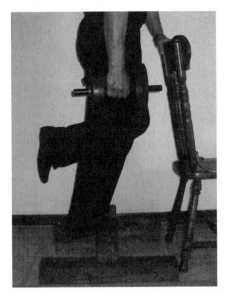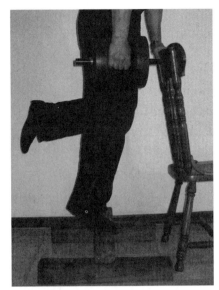

(Photo 7.27)   One-Legged Standing Calf Raises

Comments

The key to getting maximum benefit from calf raises is a full range of motion and the total time under tension. The motion should be a smooth and steady up and down.

In the up position, you should be standing as high as possible on the balls of your feet with the gastrocnemius muscle fully contracted. In the lowered position, your heels should be below the level of your toes. This low heel position provides a good stretch for the muscles and all important Achilles tendon.

The wooden block used should be high enough so that when you have lowered your heel as far as comfortably possible, the heel is still not touching the ground.

At the risk of being repetitive, I will again stress the importance of a slow, smooth, and fully controlled up-down motion. Do NOT bounce at the bottom or lower yourself too quickly. We want to tone and condition muscles, not incur tendon injuries as a result of quick, jerky, or sloppy exercise technique.

I have described a one-legged version here, as it provides for maximum stimulation while exercising. Depending on age, fitness level, and balance, some individuals may prefer using both feet at the same time for better stability.

MIDSECTION

Very few people today are happy with their midsection. This sentiment is supported by statistical trends. Reports from both the *Journal of the American Medical Association* and *Gallup-Healthways Well-Being Index* reported that over 60% of Americans are overweight or obese.

The key to a firm waist is largely based on diet. An overweight person can perform hundreds of sit-ups per day for the remainder of their lives, but they will never lose the belly and love handles if they don't clean up their diet.

You can't flex fat. The message here is that no matter how firm the stomach may be, it will never be visible if it is hidden under a blanket of excess fat. It is also important to remember that excess body fat accumulates from the inside out. This means that if you feel you are overweight around the middle, then you already have excess body fat inside your body surrounding the organs.

In recent years, the concept of training your body's core has become a popular trend. In essence, the idea here is to strengthen the entire region of the body that helps stabilize the spine and pelvis.

As an aging individual, we have similar goals. When we design an exercise regimen for our midsection, we are not only focused on the abdominal muscles but also the lower back, lower pelvic region, and lateral sides of the waist.

Exercising the midsection for people over 40 is intended to strengthen the entire region to help improve posture, maintain flexibility, minimize risks of hernia, and reduce problems associated with lower back pain.

You will perform one set of each exercise in succession. The goal is to perform 20 repetitions of each exercise, although it is to be expected that some people will only be able to perform half that many at the beginning. That is OK. We are trying to improve ourselves here. If you were already in perfect shape for your age, it is a good chance you would not be reading this book.

People already plagued with a history of lower back problems should consult with their doctor before performing most of these exercises. While all the movements shown here are time tested and well documented as excellent exercises for training the midsection, it is possible that certain individuals may have unique spinal problems that could be aggravated by repetitive waist motion.

So if you have no serious back problems and your personal physician agrees you can benefit from the program described, let's get to work on that midsection.

Crunches

Starting Position
Lie on your back with your heels resting on the surface of a bench or other flat surface. The height of this support should be such that your thighs are perpendicular to the floor. Your knees should be in an approximate 90 degree angle.

Cross your arms in front of your chest or at the sides of your head (see Photos 7.28 and 7.29).

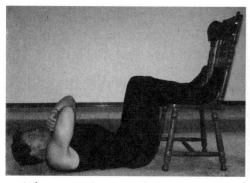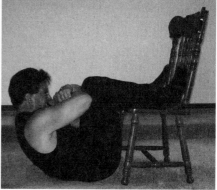

(Photo 7.28) Crunches

Movement

1. Earlier we discussed proper breathing techniques when exerting force to lift a weight. That wisdom also comes into play when exercising the midsection. When training the waist, we want to avoid building up intrathoracic pressure inside the abdomen.

2. This is achieved by being sure to exhale when crunching forward and inhaling when lying backward. Keeping this breathing rhythm in mind, slightly raise your hips off the floor, suck in your stomach slightly, while at the same time curling (crunching) your upper body forward towards your knees, effectively shortening your torso.

3. Be sure to exhale during this entire forward motion while feeling the contraction in your entire abdominal region.

Perform 1 set of 20 repetitions.

Comments

The crunch replaces the common sit up most of us did back in school. Since that time, several studies have revealed that the traditional sit up is not as effective as the crunch for targeting the abdominal region. In fact, the common sit up shifts much of the work to the hip flexors and can also aggravate lower back pain.

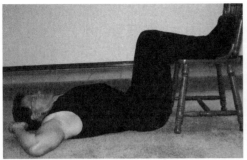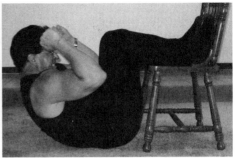

(Photo 7.29) Crunches with hands held beside head

The crunch looks like a simple exercise with a small range of motion, but it is actually a bit tricky to perform properly. In order to be totally effective, you must simultaneously raise the hips slightly, exhale your breath, curl your body forward, and vacuum your waist in slightly.

Sometimes when people first start doing this movement, they try to imitate the motion of a conventional sit up. Doing so will most likely bring the hamstrings into play. We do not want this. We want to keep all the focus and intensity on the abdominal muscles.

Don't think of sitting up as much as curling your upper body forward like the small worms you see in a springtime garden. You may need to experiment a little with the timing of your small hip lift, breathing, sucking your stomach in and curling forward, but once you do the motion properly and feel your abdominals doing all the work, you will never forget the feel.

You will then have mastered the crunch.

Leg Raises

Starting Position

Lie on your back on the floor. Form a triangle-shaped cradle with your hands and place beneath your buttocks to offer lower back support. Extend your legs straight out with your knees only slightly bent.

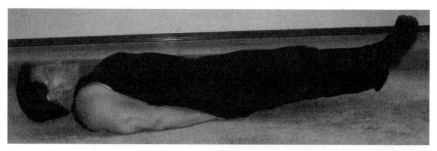

(Photo 7.30) Leg Raises

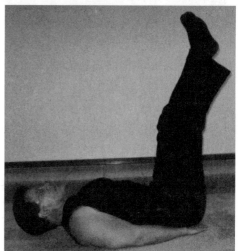

Movement

1. While exhaling, slowly raise your legs using your lower abdominal muscles until they are not quite perpendicular to the ground.

2. While inhaling, slowly lower your legs until your heels are just 1–2" off the floor. Do not allow your heels to touch the floor.

3. Once again slowly raise your legs to the top position.

4. Repeat this movement for the desired number of repetitions.

Perform 1 set of 20 repetitions.

Comments

In the movement description for this exercise, you will notice I mention that your heels should not touch the floor at any time during your repetitions. Additionally, I stress not letting your legs rise all the way to a 90 degree angle. The goal is to keep tension on the lower abdominals during the full movement and duration of the exercise. Resting the heels on the floor or raising the legs until they are a perfect 90 degree angle will take the workload off the abdominals.

Toning the lower abdominals is important but often neglected by many people who only focus on doing sit up motions. In fact, most people experience weakness and sagging of the lower abdominals with age. The lower abdominal region around the navel is where many people complain they first notice "belly bulge."

Good Mornings

Starting Position
I want to make a special cautionary note that people with a history of any type of lower back or disc problems consult their doctor before performing this exercise.

Stand upright with your feet shoulder width apart. Keep your toes pointed straight ahead. Cross your arms in front of your body.

Movement
1. While exhaling, slowly bend forward at the waist while keeping a natural arch in your lower back. Your back should not be bowing or bending during this movement. It may be helpful to imagine a yardstick taped to your back, holding it firmly in place. Also focus on keeping your legs straight through the entire motion, with no bending.

2. Bend forward until your upper torso is parallel to the floor. You should feel the work being performed by your lower back. You may also feel the hamstrings of the rear leg contributing to the effort.

3. Slowly unbend and return to an upright standing position.

Beginners may not be able to complete the desired number of repetitions of this exercise at one time. Start with as many as you can do using proper form and work up to the desired number of repetitions.

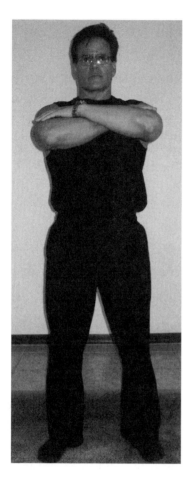

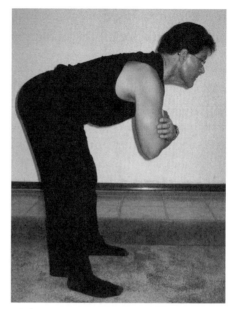

(Photo 7.31) Good Mornings

Perform 1 set of 20 repetitions.

Comments

The Good Morning movement demonstrated here is a variation of the Hyperextension exercise demonstrated in earlier chapters. In Chapter 5, I related a story of how the hyperextension has helped to virtually eliminate my own lower back problems.

Both the Good Morning and hyperextension are great exercises to strengthen the spinal erectors and may help you avoid experiencing future lower back problems. For those people who already suffer from occasional lower back issues, this movement may be beneficial in diminishing discomfort and restoring functionality.

Side Bends

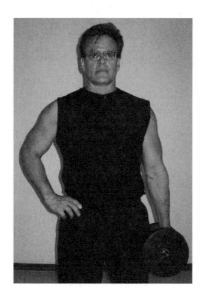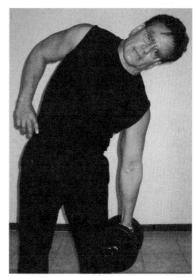

(Photo 7.32) Side Bends

Starting Position
Grab a light dumbbell in your left hand. Stand with your feet slightly less than shoulder width apart. Stand erect. Allow the weight to pull your torso downward until you feel a healthy stretch on the right side of your waist.

Movement
1. Using the strength of your right oblique muscle, straighten your torso back to a standing erect position.

Perform 1 set of 20 repetitions for each side of your body.

Comments

Be sure to only use a light weight with this exercise. The goal is to tighten and tone the lateral oblique muscles, not promote size growth.

I suggest that you alternate Side Bends and Good Morning movements with each training session. In this way, both the lower back and sides of the waist get exercised weekly.

Cardiovascular Exercise

In Chapter 5, I explained the importance and fine points of cardiovascular exercise in detail. For the sake of convenience in this chapter on home training, I have repeated much of that information below.

Your goal will be to build up to 30 minutes.

Depending on your current level of fitness, 30 minutes of continuous cardio activity may be too demanding at first. If this is the case, start with a shorter time interval of 10–15 minutes, or whatever you can handle.

30 minutes is only a duration of time. When we discuss cardiovascular exercise, we must consider both time and intensity.

How intense should the 30 minutes of cardio exercise be? 30 minutes of casually strolling around the block is far different than fast jogging for half an hour.

In order to increase cardiovascular fitness and burn excess body fat, you need to exercise within your Target Heart Rate.

What is the Target Heart Rate (THR)?

Medical researchers have established that in order to gain significant benefit from any cardiovascular related exercise, the heart rate must be elevated to a higher than normal level for at least 20 minutes.

Different sources will show some minor deviation in the upper and lower limits for suggested THR, but they are all essentially in the same ball park.

The first step in knowing your Target Heart Rate range is to calculate your Maximum Heart Rate in beats per minute. Maximum heart rate is calculated using the formula:

Maximum Heart Rate (bpm) = 220 – Your Age

Example: For a 50 year old individual.
MHR = 220 – 50 = 170 bpm

The Mayo Foundation for Medical Education and Research as well as the Center for Disease Control and Prevention utilize the values of 70% MHR and 85% MHR to determine the range you should aim for when performing vigorous cardiovascular exercise.

The CDC, as well as fitness professionals who work with rehabilitation patients and the elderly, will often aim for a milder Target Heart Range of 50% MHR to 70% MHR. This range is also desirable when working with individuals new to an exercise routine or having prior health concerns.

Continuing with our example for a 50 year old individual:

Moderate Activity Target Heart Range (50–70% of MHR)
Lower Rate Limit (bpm) = MHR x 0.50
Upper Rate Limit (bpm) = MHR x 0.70

Example: For our 50 year old test subject.
Lower Rate Limit = 170 x 0.50 = 85 bpm
Upper Rate Limit = 170 x 0.70 = 119 bpm

Vigorous Activity Target Heart Range (70–85% of MHR)
Lower Rate Limit (bpm) = MHR x 0.70
Upper Rate Limit (bpm) = MHR x 0.85

> *Example: For our 50 year old test subject.*
> *Lower Rate Limit = 170 x 0.70 = 119 bpm*
> *Upper Rate Limit = 170 x 0.85 = 145 bpm*

In the example above, we can see that a 50-year-old person aiming to perform 30 minutes of cardio exercise at a moderate intensity level should keep their heart rate between 85–119 beats per minute.

The same individual who is better conditioned, and free of any known medical conditions, may wish to perform at a more vigorous level. In this case, they would aim to maintain their heart rate between 119–145 for the full 30 minutes of cardio exercise.

The Maximum Heart Rate and subsequent target ranges are all derived from an empirical formula derived through years of research by medical professionals. While history has shown this calculation to be very accurate for the vast majority of people, it is very important that you discuss your personal health conditions with your doctor. There are a variety of medical conditions, as well as medications (such as beta blockers), that are known to have an effect on maximum heart rate.

You now know what Target Heart Range is and how it is calculated. You also understand that these theoretical ranges may need to be slightly adjusted based on your personal medical history. A personal physician can offer some guidance in regard to this issue.

For your convenience, the following chart shows these MHR and THR values for ages 30 through 105, calculated at five year intervals.

Age	Max Heart Rate-bpm	50% MHR	70% MHR	85% MHR
30	190	95	133	162
35	185	93	130	157
40	180	90	126	153
45	175	88	123	149
50	170	85	119	145
55	165	83	116	140
60	160	80	112	136
65	155	78	109	132
70	150	75	105	128
75	145	73	102	123
80	140	70	98	119
85	135	68	95	115
90	130	65	91	111
95	125	63	88	106
100	120	60	84	102
105	115	58	81	98

At the beginning of this chapter, I listed a treadmill as an optional piece of exercise equipment that the home-based trainer may wish to consider purchasing. For those who own such a treadmill, the following few pages will describe the proper use of this equipment.

Treadmill

Using the treadmill is as simple as walking. Some people may be inclined to ask the question, "Why is a treadmill any more beneficial than walking around my neighborhood?" This is a fair question. In fact, there are a number of advantages offered by the treadmill that don't always immediately come to mind.

- Despite the best of intentions, it is often hard to maintain a fast walking pace when simply taking a walk around your block or through the park. All too often our minds begin to think about other issue in our lives and before we realize it, we have slowed our walking speed down considerably. In this regard, the treadmill helps us by maintaining a set speed.

- Treadmills allow for variable resistance by offering inclines typically ranging from flat to 15 degrees. These different slopes not only change intensity but also target different walking muscles. A steep incline impacts your buttocks, calves, and hamstrings more than walking at a shallow angle. These inclines are especially useful for people living in flat terrain regions such as the Midwestern Plains and Florida where natural hills do not exist.

- Treadmills offer the ability to walk in any climate condition. Regardless of the outside weather being rainy, cold, hot, or covered in snow, you can always jump on the treadmill.

- Some people find walking to be boring, or feel they have limited time each day to squeeze in 30 minutes of cardiovascular exercise. Using a treadmill at home allows you to watch your favorite TV show or DVD while you are exercising. Almost everybody I know over the age of 40 watches at least one or two TV shows each evening. This is a perfect way to kill two birds with one stone. You still watch your favorite shows AND do something good for yourself instead of turning into a couch potato.

- Most modern treadmills feature the ability to give real time readings of your heart rate. This makes it easy to stay within your target range throughout your workout. In fact, virtually all modern treadmills feature preset programs that offer variety in intensity. Additionally, as an aid to keeping track of your progress, they also provide information such as total distance walked and calories burned.

Starting Position

Stand on the treadmill. Today, even the most affordable motorized models prompt you for time and incline. More expensive versions offer other variables such as the type of walk you desire to perform. These advanced options normally range from simple manual control of incline and speed to preprogrammed trails that emulate random walks up hills, through mountains, etc.

Movement

1. Simply walk at a brisk pace with a full natural stride.

2. Periodically monitor your heart rate and ensure you are inside your target zone.

3. Depending on your comfort level, you may either swing your arms freely as when walking naturally, or place a light hold on one of the support rails for balance.

4. As needed, adjust the incline and speed of the treadmill so that you remain inside your Target Heart Rate zone for 30 minutes.

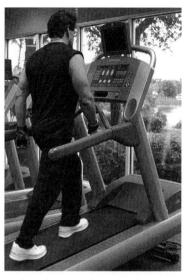

(Photo 7.33) Treadmill. In this example, incline is set to 15 degrees and speed is 2.5 mph.

Comments

In your earliest stages of walking on the treadmill, you may choose to select a fixed incline and speed which provides suitable resistance to keep you in your target heart rate range. *(For example, a 9 degree incline and speed of 3.3 mph is about right for me.)*

However, recent research has shown additional benefit is derived when the work intensity is variable over time as opposed to being a static condition. This means that instead of spending the full 30 minutes walking at an incline of 9 degrees and a speed of 3.3 and maintaining a heart rate of 130bpm, our 50-year-old test subject may periodically change the speed and incline to offer variable resistance and heart rate.

For 5 minutes, a shallow incline and quicker walking speed of 4.0 mph may be selected. Then for the next 5 minutes, the incline is ramped up to 15 degrees and the speed lowered to 2.5 mph. These kinds of variable adjustments should continue every 5 minutes for the full duration of the cardiovascular session.

During these types of changes the heart rate will of course increase and decrease to meet the demand. The important thing is to be sure you stay between the lower and upper limits of your target zone. In this example, with our 50-year-old who may be aiming for a vigorous training level, his heart rate will fluctuate between 119–145bpm throughout the 30 minute routine.

An additional benefit of this variability is that it places emphasis on different leg muscles. It will also minimize joint discomfort which sometimes occurs from repetitive identical motion.

Walking and other Options

Although I made the recommendation of a treadmill for the individual who intends to be a 100% home-based trainer, such equipment is not mandatory. Additionally, several manufacturers now offer other equipment like elliptical machines that are priced low enough for home use.

Walking outside will certainly serve as excellent cardiovascular exercise providing you are careful to pay attention to your Target Heart Rate. As I indicated earlier, the problem many people (myself included) have with fresh air walking is that they start looking at nature and tend to slow their pace. Sometimes when walking outside, the mind also begins to wander and think about work or other problems. The result is the same, the walking speed slows and the heart rate falls below the desired range for stimulating cardio fitness.

I certainly don't discourage speed walking as an option for cardiovascular exercise. I only stress the importance of paying attention to the Target Heart Rate to ensure you get the optimum benefit from your time and effort.

Looking Down the Road

The 3 day routine discussed in this chapter is by no means intended to be the final word on exercising at home. Without a doubt, if you have not been actively working to improve your fitness in the past, this routine will produce satisfying results.

Despite this, I realize with time,many people will wish to incorporate more exercises into their routine. Additionally, some individuals may want to add a fourth day of exercise into their weekly regimen.

If you participate in an active sport like tennis, open water SCUBA, biking, hiking, or the like, then you can think of a day spent doing one of these activities as a fourth day of training.

If you do not participate in any vigorous sports, but desire to add a fourth day of training, another day of cardiovascular training is an excellent option.

For people over the age of 40 or 50, many health professionals tend to agree that four days of 45 minutes duration is the maximum amount of cardiovascular training one should pursue each week.

What is the logic behind this guideline? As we all know, the aging process brings with it an increased concern over joint and connective tissue injury or wear. In the range of 3–4 days per week, 30–45 minutes per session, the body receives sufficient cardiovascular stimulation to benefit health and burn excess body fat.

However, there seems to be a point where too much consistent activity for too many days per week begins to initiate an increase in pain and fatigue in joints, tendons, and ligaments.

When older individuals begin doing more than four days of strenuous training per week, it is not uncommon to see complaints of mild pain and discomfort increase. The most probable explanation for this phenomenon is the fact that older bodies heal and recover more slowly. As a result, the best results are obtained by stimulating, but not annihilating our muscles, joints, and organs.

You Did It

You have just finished the full home training routine composed of weight resistance training, freehand movements, and cardiovascular exercise. In 12–16 weeks, combined with the diet principles you learned earlier, you will most certainly see and feel improvement in your fitness condition and energy levels.

For the sake of convenience, the following page has a summary of this routine you can photocopy and keep handy for reference while exercising until you have it memorized.

Home Training Quick Reference Guide

Perform 5-minute Warm Up routine before beginning training.
Unless otherwise noted, freehand exercises are 3 sets of 10-12 reps each.
Unless otherwise noted, dumbbell exercises are
> 1 warm-up set of 20 reps + 3 Working Sets of 12-10-8 reps.

Chest
Push-Ups

Shoulders
Dumbbell Presses OR Lateral Raises

Triceps
Chair Dips OR Overhead Extensions

Back
One Arm Dumbbell Rows

Biceps
Dumbbell Curls

Trapezius
Dumbbell Shrugs

Forearms
Forearm Curls and Spring Exerciser

Quadriceps (front of leg)
Deep Knee Bends *(10-12 reps)* and Dumbbell Squats *(10-12 reps)*

Hamstrings (back of leg)
Standing Leg Curl *(10-12 reps)*

Calves
One-Legged Standing Calf Raises *(15-20 reps)*

Midsection
Crunches and Leg Raises and (Good Mornings OR Side Bends)
1 set of 20 reps for each exercise

Cardio
Treadmill OR Brisk Speed Walking
30 minutes in Target Heart Range

Chapter Eight

Odds and Ends

Supplements, Healthy Habits, and Other Tips and Tricks That Really Work

This chapter features a collection of useful tips and information that many readers may find beneficial.

The world is a big place, and every day man's scientific and technical knowledge becomes more diverse. With each passing decade, it seems people become more specialized in their scope of knowledge. Simply stated, nobody knows it all—but with the passage of time it becomes even harder to keep up to date on everything.

You may be a wizard at car repair, and know the entire history of the automobile from 1893 to present—a respectable mass of knowledge in itself. Yet, you may have no clue how raw silicon crystals get transformed into the computer chips that serve as the "brains" of your own Smartphone or MP3 player.

Along these lines, many medical doctors I know will confess they are highly proficient at treating patients after illness or injury occur. But these same doctors will ask me questions regarding diet, exercise, and supplementation. As my own physician once told me, "In medical school, we are trained to fix the car after it has crashed. Not as much time is spent learning to prevent the crash from happening in the first place."

Certainly in recent years, medical schools have started to spend more time on diet and exercise guidelines than they did in the past, but the main focus of the medical industry is still to treat and medicate problems after they develop.

None of the information provided below should be viewed or used as a substitute for professional medical advice, diagnosis, counseling or treatment. Instead, what follows should be seen as a collection of tips and tricks that have proven beneficial to many people, and may help you too.

WAKING BED STRETCHES

When you were 10 years old, you could jump out of bed and hit the ground running. Unless you were careless enough to run into a wall, discomfort was not even in your mind. 40 years later, jumping out of bed is probably not quite as trouble free as it was back then.

Chances are if you are like most people over 40, the first few steps of the morning bring some cracks and pops along with random joint pain. For many older people, the first 30 minutes of the morning means soreness in the feet, arches, ankles, knees, or lower back. Others may have shoulder, elbow, hand, or even neck pains.

When we sleep, connective tissue and muscles stiffen. Quite often we sleep in a bad position that can throw joints out of perfect alignment.

Spending just 3–5 minutes performing a few stretches in bed before putting your feet on the floor works wonders to make the early morning more pleasant.

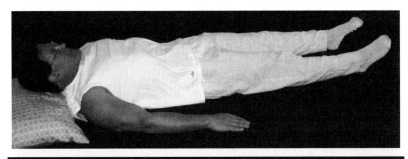

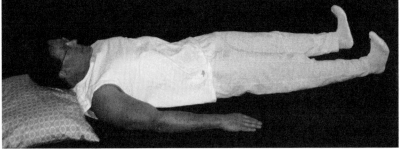

(Photo 8.1) Calf Stretch & Ankle Rotations

Calf Stretch & Ankle Rotations

Starting Position
Lie flat on your back in bed.

Movement
1. With your legs straight and resting on the bed, move your toes upwards and downwards as far as possible in a slow stretching motion. This movement is identical to the calf raise exercise you learned earlier.

2. After 5–10 stretches, slowly rotate your ankles both clockwise and counterclockwise.

3. Finish off with 5–10 more "calf raise" stretching motions.

Comments

This morning stretch is often beneficial to people who have problems with their ankles when they take their first few steps each morning.

Knee Ups

Starting Position

Lie flat on your back in bed.

Movement

1. Slowly bend your right leg, pulling it up to your chest. Gently hug your folded knee, while allowing your lower back to stretch.

2. Slowly allow your leg to straighten. When the leg is straightened, tense the frontal thigh muscles near the knee.

3. Repeat at least 5 times or until your lower back feels better.

4. Perform the same movement for your left leg.

Comments

This stretch is an in-bed variation of a stretching motion often recommended for individuals with lower back problems.

I have several friends and associates who have varying degrees of back problems. This morning stretch combined with the one that follows has

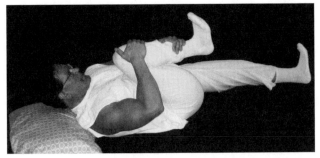

(Photo 8.2) Knee Ups

helped them alleviate the random twinges they used to get when first moving around in the morning.

As an added bonus, this movement also gets the knees loose and ready to walk after a full night's sleep.

Buttocks Squeeze & Lower Back Tense

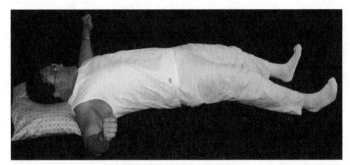

(Photo 8.3) Buttocks Squeeze & Lower Back Tense

Starting Position
Lie flat on your back in bed.

Movement
1. While lying flat on the bed, squeeze your buttocks muscles while at the same time tensing your lower back and pressing your rear shoulders into the bed. The motion is similar to a soldier being told to "stand at attention" —but in this case, you are lying down.

When properly performed, you should feel a slight arch in your back as your midsection rises slightly upwards toward the ceiling. At this same time, it will feel as though your shoulders and heels are supporting a larger percentage of your bodyweight.

5 of these should do the trick.

Comments

Those individuals who are plagued with recurring back spasms or other lower back problems may find it useful to alternate between this stretching motion and the previous one.

Arm & Elbow Stretches

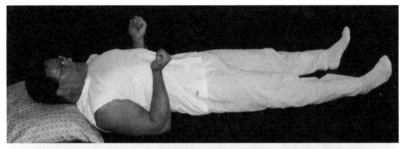

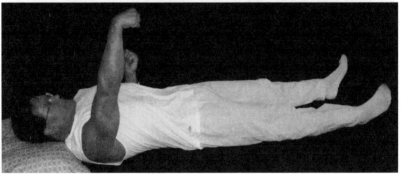

(Photo 8.4) The benefit of this warm up movement exists in the subtle details regarding elbow and wrist motion.

Starting Position

Lie flat on your back with your arms and hands positioned as shown in the photo above. You should have your wrists bent backwards as far as comfortable such that you feel a mild stretch in the wrists and forearms.

Movement

1. Slowly extend your right arm forward as though you are throwing a punch in slow motion. As your hand moves forward, rotate your wrist so that when you reach full extension, your fist is in a palm downward position.

2. Hold this extended position as you tilt your wrist forward and downward toward the opposing wall. You should feel a nice stretch along the top of your forearm extending all the way back to your outer elbow region.

3. Reverse the motion, bringing your arm back to the starting position. You should also rotate your wrists so that by the time your arms are withdrawn, your hands are also in the starting position. Repeat for the left arm.

4. Continue until you have done 5–10 of these for each arm.

Comments

The key to getting benefit from this motion is to ensure the wrists are flexed as far as possible until you can feel the gentle stretch extending along the forearm from the wrist to the elbows. This motion is similar to a common therapy exercise for people suffering from tendonitis.

Wrist Rotations

Starting Position

Lie on your back with your elbows bent at a 90 degree angle and your hands in front of your body.

Movement

1. This movement is very simple. Just rotate both wrists clockwise for 5–10 repetitions. Repeat in the opposite direction. Most people

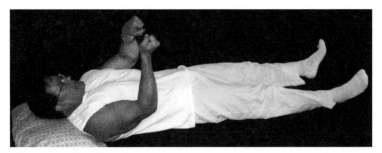

(Photo 8.5) Wrist Rotations.

find it easier to rotate the wrists in an opposite mirror image of each other.

Comments

This is a very simple motion, but it can be very beneficial to prevent injury. With age, some people complain that their wrists and ankles "get hung up" or otherwise click and pop when working under a load.

Three Part Hand and Finger Stretch

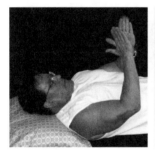 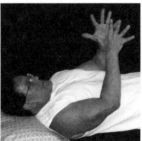 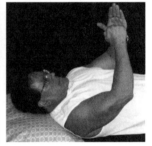

(Photo 8.6) Three Part Hand and Finger Stretch

Starting Position

Lie on your back with your elbows bent at a 90 degree angle and your hands in front of your body.

Movement

1. Start by holding your hands flat with your fingers together. At this point, your hands should be in a posture that you see in classic karate movies.

2. Slowly arch the fingers of each hand backwards as far as possible using only their own muscular strength. You should feel the tension along the tendons on the back of the fingers and hand.

3. Allow your hands to return to the "karate" position. Now fan your fingers out as wide as possible.

4. Return to the karate position and close your hands to form a fist.

5. Depending on the amount of finger or joint pain that normally exists in the morning, 5–10 repetitions should be all that is needed to get the finger joints loose and comfortable.

Comments

This is a simple motion, but it can be very beneficial to people who have suffered extensor tendon injury (mallet finger) or other hand injuries. Often such individuals have problems with these past injuries causing joints to stiffen or feel out of joint upon waking in the morning.

Shrug and Neck Stretch

Starting Position

Sit upright in place or sit on the edge of your bed with feet flat on the floor. Choose the position you find most comfortable.

Movement

1. Slowly and fully pull your shoulders straight upwards in a shrugging motion similar to that made when saying "I don't know."

2. Slowly lower your shoulders back to their natural position.

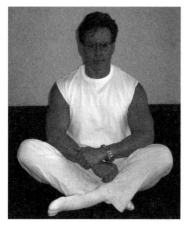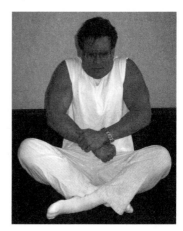

(Photo 8.7) Shrug and Neck Stretch

3. Repeat for 5–10 repetitions or until your neck and shoulder region feels loose and comfortable.

Comments

Like all the stretching motions described here, these shrugs are quick and easy to perform. Despite their simplicity, they can work wonders to help a shoulder or neck that has spent eight hours lying in a bad position.

Okay, that is it for the waking bed stretches. Now, head out to the kitchen and start your day.

Drink a Glass of Water First Thing upon Waking

In Chapter 3 we summarized some benefits to distilling your own water at home. If you followed up on that advice, early morning is a great time to drink that first glass of water for the day.

While we are asleep, the body works to restore itself from the day's activities. If you are now actively weight training and performing cardio then nutrients and water are being increasingly used to build muscle fibers, improve bone density, and perform basic cellular and biological functions. Water is required for almost every restoration function in the body.

Summarizing the above in fewer words, we get dehydrated while we sleep at night. Even a small degree of dehydration in the body can make you feel more tired, weaken muscular contraction strength, and adversely affect concentration. Drinking a glass of water first thing in the morning "primes" the system, restores water lost to cellular activity during the night, and helps lubricate the digestive system to prepare for the first meal of the day.

Get 15 Minutes of Sunlight Several Days per Week

Scientists have often stated that immortality will forever elude man due to a paradox created by God (or nature—depending on your personal beliefs).

The human body requires oxygen to survive. Without it, the body dies within minutes. Ironically however, the very oxygen needed to keep us alive also oxidizes the cells and forms free radicals. These free radicals cause cellular damage over time. Some researchers feel this "cellular rusting" is a major cause of the aging process. One could say the very oxygen we need to survive also slowly kills us.

A similar paradox exists with sunlight exposure. We all know excess exposure to the sun causes skin damage, wrinkling, and even the increased probability of cancer. At the same time, a lack of exposure to sunlight can cause its own problems.

Vitamin D is produced when the skin is exposed to the sun. A lack of sunlight can result in lower vitamin D levels. A lack of vitamin D can lead to muscle and joint pain. A correlation has also been established between vitamin D deficiency and increased risk of heart attack and other cardiac problems. Some studies also reveal a possible connection to multiple sclerosis.

Seasonal Affective Disorder (SAD) is a form of depression experienced by many people during the winter months. SAD is not as prevalent in tropical regions, but is seen with increased frequency by people living in the cooler Northern climates. When the days get shorter, darker, and colder, the incidence of SAD becomes more common.

Symptoms include oversleeping, less energy, fatigue, overeating, mood swings, anxiety, lowered sex drive, and difficulty with mental concentration. In most cases, SAD symptoms begin to disappear with the arrival of spring, warmer weather, and increased exposure to sunlight.

If too much sun damages our skin and increases the risk of cancer, but too little sunlight produces vitamin D deficiency and depression —what are we to do? Ideally, the goal is to get the right amount of sun to serve our biological needs and keep us healthy, while avoiding the excessive exposure that can cause harm.

For fair skinned people, many health professionals and researchers now feel 10–15 minutes of sun exposure, at least 3–4 days per week, is the optimum amount of sunlight exposure. Darker skinned individuals may require 20–30 minutes. Very dark skinned individuals will normally require as much as 45–60 minutes of sun exposure, also 3–4 days per week. Darker skinned individuals require more sunlight for vitamin D synthesis due to the protective UV-B blocking action resulting from extra pigmentation.

Ideally this sun exposure should not be during the hottest and most UV intensive hours of midday. Also these time estimates assume at least 15–30% of bare skin is exposed to the sun.

For most people, it is also worth considering supplementation with vitamin D3. 1000 IU of vitamin D3 daily is a common dosage for most adults.

Hand Sanitizer

The average person gets 2–4 colds and/or sore throats per year.
It is estimated that more people get sick from physical contact with contaminated surfaces than they do from inhaling viruses from the air.

Think about your typical day moving around in modern society.
Every day you touch door handles, public restroom faucets, gasoline dispensers, shopping carts, products on shelves, utensils at restaurants, books, computer keyboards, light switches, and hundreds of other surfaces. How many other people touched those same surfaces in the past 48 hours? How many of those individuals may have been sick with a cold, flu, or sore throat?

Many years ago, I was told that faithful use of a hand sanitizer containing a minimum of 65% ethanol could greatly reduce my own suffering from frequent colds and sore throats. Like most people, I used to experience the average 2–4 colds or sore throats per year.

I started carrying a bottle of hand sanitizer in the door pocket of my car. Anytime I am in public, the very first thing I do when getting back in my car is to apply sanitizer and work my hands together.

Knowing the cold-causing rhinovirus (and some other bugs) invades the mucous membranes inside the nose, I also gently inhale some of the alcohol vapor into my nose while the sanitizer is still wet on my hands. The idea being that this nasal disinfection might help knock out recently acquired microbes before they can get anchored and begin their devious reproduction and the resulting illness.

Has this health habit been effective? I have not had a cold or even a sore throat in the past three years. So it seems there may in fact be real benefit to this practice.

I feel to be truly effective in helping to prevent illness, this practice needs to be followed in an almost religious manner. Like clockwork, you must use the sanitizer every time you enter your car after being exposed to public surfaces. Fate is an unfaithful mistress.

Bad luck being what it is, no doubt the one time you forget this sanitizing procedure will be the same day you come into contact with contagious germs.

For those who also wish to try the slight nasal inhalation of the sanitizer vapor, I advise you to use common sense and caution. You only want to inhale a small amount of the sanitizer solution that is located just outside the openings of the nostrils. As you may expect, inhaling too much vapor can create a burning sensation in the nose.

If you suffer from frequent colds or sore throats, this may be a tip that can prove helpful in making your life more illness-free.

Low Testosterone

In recent years, advertisements for supplemental male hormone (testosterone) have increased exponentially. Most commonly, the remedy being described involves the use of a testosterone-containing cream or gel to replace what the body is not producing on its own.

As discussed in Chapter 2, there is no question that testosterone begins to decline in men after the age of 35–40. It might seem obvious that the only way to correct a lowered testosterone level is to administer an external supplemental supply of the hormone to restore the proper levels in the body.

Seems logical, right? Well, not so fast. The modern pharmaceutical mindset is to immediately begin prescribing testosterone gel for men with lowered values. The fact is, not all patients with lowered testosterone levels actually need this medical treatment to restore normal levels of the hormone.

I will relate another personal experience. The natural range for testosterone in adult males is approximately 250–1000 ng/dl. In my earlier years, my own testosterone value averaged 800 ng/dl.

When I was in my late 40s, I began to notice it became harder to maintain muscle size and strength. At the same time, it became easier to gain a few pounds of fat if I became a bit sloppy with my eating. Additionally, I noticed that occasionally I would feel a small wave of anxiety or nervousness for no apparent reason. Although nothing major, these small incidents of unexplained nervousness really grabbed my attention as I had always been fearless and worry-free until then.

At age 48, I requested my doctor to perform a full blood work profile. When the results came back, I was unpleasantly surprised to learn my testosterone value was 418 ng/dl. While this concentration was still well inside the normal range, it was a sizeable decline from the levels I possessed 20 years earlier.

My doctor explained that normally men do not experience any serious symptoms until their hormone level drops below 250 ng/dl. He lightheartedly told me, "You are experiencing the first early signs of aging."

Between ages 48–49, I repeated the same type of testing and ended up with testosterone values that ranged from 391–410 ng/dl. I did not experience any other new symptoms during this time, but it still concerned me that my levels had dropped nearly 50% compared to years earlier.

My doctor suggested I consider testosterone cream if I wanted to raise my levels. I was reluctant. I was not yet 50 years old.

I also knew that once you begin taking a hormone externally, you essentially shut down what remains of your body's own production capability. You become totally reliant on the externally administered product to maintain your hormone levels.

I decided to consult an endocrinologist for a second opinion. This second doctor who specialized specifically in endocrine function suggested I try a few supplements and clothing changes before giving up on my own body's hormone producing capabilities.

These suggestions included the following:

- Eat several servings of broccoli or cauliflower daily
- Supplemental zinc via ZMA tablets at bedtime
- Resveratrol supplementation
- Deer Velvet Antler (IGF-1) supplementation
- Tribulus terrestris supplementation
- d-Aspartic acid supplementation
- Saw Palmetto supplementation
- Avoid eating grapefruit
- Wear boxer shorts instead of tight fitting brief-style underwear
- Lose as much excess body fat as possible around the middle
- Use moderately heavy weights when performing large compound exercises like Bench Press, Leg Press, and Seated Rowing motions.

Admittedly I was skeptical that these simple, natural lifestyle changes would have any effect on my testosterone levels. However, I learned many years ago that unless something is totally insane or risky, it is worth giving it a try before passing judgment.

We agreed I would immediately make these changes. I would then get blood tests at 6, 9, and 12 weeks afterwards to see if there was any change from the hormone levels I had been exhibiting over the previous two years.

I was in for a surprise. The results for my next three blood tests were 674, 775, and 703 ng/dl total testosterone. The bio-available free testosterone was also much improved.

How could these few supplements, diet, and clothing changes increase my testosterone by 300 units? Once I learned there are two commonly recognized endocrine disorders that cause men to have lowered levels of testosterone, I was better able to understand why this natural option helped my 49-year-old body.

Two Major Reasons Men Lose Testosterone

The male hormone system can be viewed as being similar to a factory. A boss sends orders down to the factory telling it how much testosterone needs to be produced. The factory is found in the Leydig cells of the testes. The boss is the pituitary gland. The orders that are sent from the boss to the factory are lutenizing hormone (LH) and follicle stimulating hormone (FSH).

The hypothalamus portion of the brain serves as a monitor to keep check on the level of hormones in the blood. The hypothalamus and pituitary gland work together as a team.

In the case of testosterone, when the hypothalamus detects a low level in the blood, it generates a brief surge of hormone called gonadotropin-releasing hormone, which serves as a signal to the pituitary. This signal stimulates the pituitary to secrete more LH and FSH. When the Leydig cells in the testes see these higher levels of LH and FSH, they kick into production mode to manufacture more testosterone. The whole process is essentially a feedback system.

There are two primary reasons this process falters in men as they experience a decline in male hormone with age.

Primary Hypogonadism

In the first case, the Leydig cells of the testes have lost the ability to produce adequate testosterone. The hypothalamus will detect low levels of testosterone in the blood and send signals to the pituitary that the factory needs to pump up production. The pituitary will generate more and more LH and FSH as it "screams" at the Leydig cells to produce more hormones.

However, all these attempts to stimulate activity are to no avail. In this case, one could say the factory is simply worn out. No matter how much they are stimulated, the testes simply can not produce testosterone as they did years earlier.

Blood tests can reveal this condition. If a patient has very high levels of LH and FSH, but low testosterone, it usually indicates a classic case of testicular failure. The body is trying to increase production, but it is unable to do so.

For individuals who fit the above description, supplemental testosterone in the form of creams, gels, or injections is typically the only way to restore normal male hormone levels. This cause of testosterone deficiency is primarily seen in men over the age of 55.

Secondary Hypogonadism
As a general rule, most men under the age of 55 still have the potential ability to generate sufficient testosterone naturally. The "factory" is usually still alive and kicking, but there is another problem in the process.

In this second case, the testes receive little or no message from the pituitary. The Leydig cells still have the ability to produce testosterone if urged to do so, but they are not receiving the LH and FSH signals that tell them to start working.

It is not clear why this breakdown in communication between the hypothalamus-pituitary-Leydig cells occurs. Some researchers indicate possible causes ranging from damage due to viral infections, autoimmune responses, or even drug interactions.

Blood tests can also reveal this condition. If a patient has low levels of LH and FSH along with low testosterone, it usually indicates the body is not even making an effort to stimulate increased production.

The positive thing about secondary hypogonadism is that it is usually treatable. In minor cases, the synergistic effect of some simple lifestyle changes can be enough to adequately trigger natural production. In more severe cases, chorionic gonadotropin (CG) can be prescribed to essentially jump start the process and stimulate more testicular production.

So Knowing All This, Why Did a Few Supplements and Dietary Changes Help Me?

Knowing how and why testosterone levels decline with age, it is now easier to understand how the tips suggested by the endocrinologist were beneficial.

The levels of the female hormone estrogen increase with added body fat. In men, this battle between estrogen and testosterone can create a hormonal balance problem. Cruciferous vegetables like broccoli and cauliflower have anti-estrogen properties that help stimulate the burning off of extra estrogen in men.

Since I personally find it tiring to eat broccoli all the time, I also relied on dried vegetable capsules that are available from health food stores. This supplement makes it much easier to get 3–4 servings of cruciferous vegetables each day.

Grapefruit, on the other hand, tends to inhibit the liver's breakdown of estrogen.

Supplements like ZMA, Tribulus, and d-aspartic acid are all purported to increase testosterone levels. To be fair, research studies on these supplements have shown mixed results. While some results have shown no positive effects, others have shown 10–30% increases of testosterone in test subjects.

Saw Palmetto has a good reputation of inhibiting 5-alpha-reductase conversion of testosterone to DHT, and is believed by many to be beneficial in warding off prostate problems.

Interestingly enough, there also appears to be truth behind the old adage that "boxers are better than briefs" in terms of male virility. Scientists still debate this issue, but an increasing number of studies and patient feedback supports the idea that something about tight fitting underwear tends to inhibit both testosterone and sperm production in some men.

Using heavier weights when performing compound lifting motions involving large body parts has also been shown to raise testosterone levels as the body attempts to trigger its muscle growth adaption mechanism.

As I said earlier, I was totally taken by surprise when this little regimen helped me. I suspect none of these things alone would make a big difference, but in combination, the results were considerable. It has now been over a year since I first met with the endocrinologist. I just recently had blood work performed again while writing this book. My testosterone level is still close to 700 ng/dl.

The point of relating my personal story is this: if you find yourself facing a similar situation where your testosterone level has declined with age, it may be worth investigating your options.

Most family physicians will immediately suggest testosterone gels or creams as an answer. Depending on your personal situation, there may be a more natural alternative to try first before committing yourself to external hormone replacement therapy.

Prostate Health

Some enlargement of the prostate by the age of 50 can be expected by 50% of men. This figure increases to 80% by the age of 80 years old.

Most men are no doubt aware of the importance of annual physical exams of the prostate gland combined with PSA testing to try to detect health problems before they occur. This diligence becomes even more critical after the age of 40.

I am personally a firm believer in the positive benefits of Saw Palmetto supplementation for men over age 35. Typical dosages are usually 320–640 mg per day. A high quality product should be standardized to contain 85–95% free fatty acids and biologically active sterols.

As is the case with many supplements, you will find an equal number of studies that support the benefits of Saw Palmetto as those that claim it offers no positive effects at all. In either case, the reported claims for Saw Palmetto are only for helping to prevent prostate enlargement. Even the majority of Saw Palmetto advocates tend to agree this supplement offers no real benefit for treating an existing condition.

Saw Palmetto should be viewed as something you can consider for trying to prevent a problem as opposed to fixing a problem you already have. It most certainly should not be viewed as a substitute for medical treatment of a serious existing condition.

Female Hormone Stability

In the years leading up to menopause, the female body's normal levels of estrogen and progesterone begin to fluctuate in an irregular fashion. Some medical professionals use the analogy of an engine beginning to sputter in the last few minutes before it shuts down.

Because of these hormonal changes, most women experience a number of symptoms during this time. Most women experience these symptoms of perimenopause and premenopause between the ages of 43–55.

The most commonly reported symptoms include the following:

Mood changes
Irritability, impatience, or increased risks of depression are sometimes experienced during this time. A woman may realize she is not responding normally to minor life stresses, yet still struggle with her feelings and reactions.

Hot flashes and sleep problems

Approximately 70% of women experience hot flashes. This classic symptom usually occurs during late perimenopause. Women report a wide range of variation in the duration, frequency, and intensity of these symptoms.

"Night sweats" can introduce sleep problems in women who have never had problems sleeping through the night before. Even individuals who don't suffer from serious hot flashes may still notice a change in their sleeping patterns. Difficulty getting to sleep, as well as waking much earlier than desired, is a frequent problem for women during this time.

Decreasing fertility

Since menopause itself is essentially the transition point where a woman is no longer fertile and capable of reproduction, it stands to reason the ability to conceive decreases during this time.

As long as a woman is having periods, pregnancy remains a possibility. However, with ovulation becoming more erratic as the body begins to "gear down" during this time, the ability to conceive likewise diminishes.

Menstrual irregularity

Ovulation becomes erratic during this time. The time intervals between periods can be longer, shorter, or skipped altogether.

Vaginal and bladder problems

As estrogen levels decline, the vaginal tissues lose both lubrication ability and elasticity. Loss of muscle tissue tone may also introduce problems with frequent urination and/or urinary incontinence.

Changes in sexual function

During perimenopause, sexual arousal may decline. Medical professionals debate the true cause of lessened interest in sexual activity in the aging female. Some researchers believe hormonal change is the underlying culprit. Other researchers contend that testosterone more so than estrogen is the "aggressive" hormone that ignites desire. These researchers theorize self-perception, attitude, and other mental aspects have more to do with libido changes than do estrogen declines.

This latter group of researchers point to studies that reveal women with active and healthy sex lives prior to the perimenopausal years usually continue to be sexually active even after menopause.

Loss of bone
Although both men and women suffer from bone loss with age, women are more prone to osteoporosis. The rate of bone loss is proportional to the decline of estrogen in women. It is for this reason you will see so many advertisements for Calcium and Vitamin D aimed at women.

Changing cholesterol levels
Although not commonly known, the decline of estrogen can also change the relative ratios of blood cholesterol levels. With lower estrogen, it is common to see an increase in the unhealthy low-density lipoproteins (LDL). Likewise, the healthy high-density lipoproteins (HDL) levels often decrease.

This change helps to explain why heart attacks become more common in older women. When younger, men tend to demonstrate a statistically higher rate of heart disease and strokes than women of the same age. After menopause, there is less discrimination in the frequency of cardiovascular illness between older men and women.

As is the case with men, some women look to hormone replacement therapy in later life. Although a full discussion of Hormone Replacement Therapy (HRT) is worthy of its own book, there are a few things worth mentioning here.

In the past, HRT received a bad reputation for increasing the incidence of certain health issues. During this time, hormones were often introduced into the body at excessive levels, or in improper ratios to other compounds like aromatizing agents.

However, the sophistication of professionally monitored HRT treatment has improved in recent years. The goal of responsible HRT is simply to restore hormone balances to normal healthy values that alleviate some of the ill effects of old age. As with any form of medical treatment, some risks still exist.

The incidence of risk is usually connected to heredity and personal health history. The decision to pursue HRT treatment is a personal choice. In any event, it is advisable to research the benefits versus risks of this medical treatment before considering it for your own situation.

In the previous section, I recounted a personal story of how supplementation and some lifestyle changes helped me as a male offset the natural decline of testosterone.

A similar potential remedy exists for many women. The following list of supplements has proven popular in recent years. Many women claim products containing these compounds help alleviate many of the unpleasant symptoms described above—symptoms which are normally linked and attributed to the premenopausal years.

- Diindolylmethane (DIM)
- Vitamin E
- Natural phytoestrogene & natural progesterone USP

DIM is the main ingredient found in most of the health food supplements now advertised to help support a healthy balance of hormones in women. Research has shown that DIM seems to work as an estrogen balancer. By balancing estrogen and minimizing the excess accumulation of estradiol, DIM is also believed to help offset symptoms such as easier weight gain, moodiness, and breast pain.

Natural phytoestrogene and natural progesterone USP are found in a number of special purpose lotions. These formulations claim to help the body maintain a healthy estrogen/progesterone balance and ward off estrogen dominance.

As with many natural remedies, you will find an equal number of supporters and detractors to the benefits of the above supplements. Thousands, if not millions, of women attest to the benefits of these products in helping improve their quality of life. Likewise, many researchers in the medical arena will say insufficient evidence exists to confirm the benefits of these compounds. This may be a case where you will need to reach your own conclusions based on personal experience.

Bone Health

It is no secret that bone loss and osteoporosis is a common ailment for both men and women over the age of 40. Although unique hormonal changes and physiology make osteoporosis a bigger problem for women, both sexes should take the risk of bone loss seriously.

Unless there is a specific medical condition that prevents a person from taking supplemental Calcium and Vitamin D, it is pretty much universally agreed that older individuals should be taking these daily.

A regimen is as follows:

- Calcium (as Calcium Citrate)   1,000–1,200 mg/daily
- Vitamin D3   600–1,000 I.U. daily
- Sunlight exposure as detailed earlier in this chapter.

As with all the training routines and supplementation suggestions in this book, you should discuss your own personal needs with a family physician.

Joint Health

In Chapter 2, we summarized the effects age has on our joints. Aches and pains become more common in the knees, elbows, ankles, shoulders, and wrists after age 40.

Many people will attest to the benefits of Glucosamine-Chondroitin-MSM supplementation in helping to maintain healthy joints and connective tissue. A common formulation of these supplements will look as follows when you read the label:

- Glucosamine (sulfate)   750 mg
- Chondroitin (sulfate)   600 mg
- Methylsulfonylmethane (MSM)   500 mg

Eye Health

As the eyes age, they lose the ability to focus over a wide range of distances. Aging eyes also lose nutrients essential for health. This lost of nutrients is thought to make problems like macular degeneration and cataracts more probable.

In recent years, products have been introduced that seem to show positive benefits in helping to maintain healthy eyes. These products normally contain the following ingredients:

- Lutein
- Zeaxanthin
- Omega-3 fatty acids
- Vitamins A, C, E
- Minerals: Zinc, Selenium, Copper

Cholesterol Control

Occasionally when a patient first begins to exhibit high cholesterol values, their family doctor may suggest diet and lifestyle changes before prescribing a medication. This is particularly the case when that patient's cholesterol values are only slightly elevated.

The normal rule of thumb is that Total Cholesterol is best maintained at levels lower than 200 mg/dl. In the range of 201–239 mg/dl, family physicians often try to get their patients to lower their cholesterol values through natural means. When total cholesterol exceeds 240 mg/dl, physicians become more inclined to suggest prescription medications.

Some individuals who only need to lower their cholesterol slightly have had positive results from the following:

- Eat oatmeal for breakfast.
- Reduce intake of high cholesterol foods like shrimp, fast foods, deep fried food, egg yolks, etc.
- Exercise regularly
- Lose weight if carrying excess body fat
- No smoking
- Increase fiber intake in the daily diet
- Niacin (Flush-free) Supplementation   500 mg/daily

While it would not be advisable for an existing patient to stop taking cholesterol medicine without a doctor's advice, the suggestions above may prove useful to many readers. Suppose your last annual physical revealed that your total cholesterol was 212 mg/dl. Some of these ideas may be worth trying.

If you are now facing a cholesterol value that is only slightly elevated, discuss the information above with your doctor. Maybe these small changes can help you too, and prevent the need to begin taking medication.

Wash Cooked Meat to Reduce Fat and Calories

Earlier I explained that many people grew up learning a style of cooking that relies heavily on fat, salt, and pepper for flavoring. Only in the past few decades has increased travel and more cultural diversity made people familiar with exotic foods.

In my own case, growing up in Virginia during the 60s and 70s, all the local restaurants were traditional American fare of steaks, potatoes, macaroni and cheese, green beans, apple pie, and buttered bread. At home, my grandparents and mother primarily relied on "country cooking" recipes that derived from the Old World.

Asian, Indian, and Mexican foods, for example, were almost unheard of. It was not until I moved to South Florida in the 80s that I first experienced Thai food and other foreign dishes. Of course, our society has changed quite a bit in the past 40 years, and today even the smallest towns across America seem to have a variety of culinary choices ranging from Chinese, Thai, Mexican, Cuban, Ethiopian, Indian, Korean, Japanese, Vietnamese, Peruvian, etc.

Why do I mention this? The introduction of these well-seasoned dishes has taught us that fats, salt, and pepper are not the only way to make food taste good. The skilled use of herbs and spices can often offer more powerful flavor than fats and salt alone.

One useful trick for reducing fat and calories in your favorite meat dishes is to wash the cooked meat before final preparation. Take tacos for example. When the ground beef is almost fully cooked, you can remove the deep skillet from the heat and add several cups of water. Depending on your wrist and arm strength you can either tilt the skillet to rinse the meat 1–2 times with water , or, you can pour the water and cooked meat mixture into a fine mesh strainer.

Regardless of the technique used, the objective is to wash all the greasy fat off the meat. Once drained, the washed meat can now be returned to the skillet to complete preparation.

I know there are a number of you who will at first think removing all this greasy fat will make the meat tasteless. However, with the proper use of taco seasoning, hot sauce, liquid smoke, and other seasonings you can actually have tacos that taste great (not just fatty and greasy).

The big advantage to this little trick is that depending on the cut and type of meat being prepared, fat and calorie content can be reduced by as much as 30%. I actually use this technique all the time when preparing meats. After a lifetime of eating greasy, fatty hamburger this may seem a little strange at first, but you will almost certainly end up liking it better. In time the sight, smell, and taste of cooked meat swimming in a puddle of greasy fat will probably become nauseating.

A similar phenomenon is sometimes seen with people who switch to 100% natural peanut butter. At first, these folks usually find the natural peanut butter strange. But after a time, most people begin to prefer the taste of the real thing. In fact, it soon becomes almost impossible to eat the popular name brands that are loaded with sugar, hydrogenated oils, and other fillers. That type of peanut butter will soon taste cheap, fake, too sweet, and synthetic by comparison to the 100% natural stuff.

Depression and Anxiety

Almost 12% of Americans take some form of medication for depression. Worldwide, the pharmaceutical sales of antidepressant medications now exceed $20 billion per year. Most alarming is a recent report that disclosed antidepressant use has skyrocketed 400% since the late 1980s.

What has changed over the past 30 years? Are people less happy today, or, have we developed an overreliance on pills in our modern society?

Depression and anxiety can be very serious problems for those who suffer from these conditions. It is far beyond the scope of this book to discuss this topic in any depth. I do however wish to make you aware of research and case studies conducted by Doctor Stephen S. Ilardi, PhD.

In his book *The Depression Cure*, Dr. Ilardi outlines a 6-step program he has used in his own practice. Among his study patients, the rate of favorable response has been substantially greater than that seen with people who only follow a traditional antidepressant medication treatment.

Briefly summarized, Dr. Ilardi's treatment includes the following:

- Omega-3 supplementation (1000mg EPA / 500mg DHA daily)
- Vitamin D supplementation (2000 IU daily)
- Multivitamin supplementation
- Vitamin C (500 mg daily)
- Evening Primrose Oil (500 mg weekly)
- Sunlight Exposure
- Vigorous Physical Exercise at least 3 days per week
- Positive Socialization
- Adequate Sleep
- Learning to Break the Internal Mental Rumination Cycle
- Engage in distracting activities that force mental concentration

In addition to the suggestions offered above, other supplements that have proven beneficial to many individuals dealing with mild depression, panic attacks, and anxiety include:

- St. Johns Wort
- SAM-e
- L-Theanine

I would never encourage a person suffering from depression and anxiety to avoid professional medical treatment. I only make mention of this research and its promising results for those who may wish to further investigate possible options.

For the individual just experiencing their first minor waves of anxiety or depression, various lifestyle changes may prove helpful. For people who feel that medication alone is not helping them with their existing conditions, there might be some helpful information to be discovered by reading the works of doctors and researchers like Dr. Ilardi.

I would encourage any of you currently dealing with depression or anxiety issues to discuss these ideas with your own doctor to see if a synergistic approach might prove more effective.

There is one last consideration to keep in mind. Supplements like St. Johns Wort can cause interactions with some prescription medications. Likewise, St. Johns Wort is also known to increase sensitivity to sunlight. For this reason, it is advisable to fully research any new supplement you may wish to include in your daily regimen. Although a certain supplement may have a good track record for helping others, your own allergies and medical history could produce different results.

Don't Eat in the Three Hours Prior to Bedtime

There are several benefits to not eating in the three hours prior to going to bed for the night:

- Easier to fall asleep
- Help prevent excess weight gain
- Minimize problems with gastric reflux and heartburn
- Aid in preventing a "sour stomach" the next morning

When you go to bed with a full stomach, it sets the stage for several undesirable effects. The heat generated from the digestion process makes it more difficult for some people's bodies to "gear down" and prepare for sleep.

The average person sleeps more soundly in a slightly cooled condition. This is one reason many professionals suggest bedroom thermostats be set around 62–72 degrees.

Digestion of heavy meals at this late hour can also interfere with the generation of melatonin, a neurohormone that aids in proper sleep.

If you recall our earlier discussion on calorie utilization and the body's natural tendency to digest and process food in 3–4 hour windows, the disadvantage of bedtime eating is self evident. Excess calories consumed just prior to eight hours of sleep and relative inactivity are more prone to be converted to body fat.

The simple law of gravity explains why going to bed with a full stomach can worsen gastric reflux and other stomach problems. Lying down after a full meal will naturally cause more stomach contents to try to flow backward (and upward) through the esophageal valve at the top of the stomach.

Being new to healthier and lighter eating, are you struggling with hunger pangs? After 10, 20, or 30 years of heavy eating it is understandable your body will go through some withdrawal symptoms in the first few weeks after changing your eating habits.

Hunger urges normally come in waves, and last 10–15 minutes. One of the best ways to offset the desire to eat in the hours before bedtime is to drink a glass of water when you feel hungry. The physical volume of water is usually sufficient to nullify the hunger urges more rapidly.

If you are able to resist the urge to snack late at night, you will usually find the hunger instinct will pass in a quarter of an hour. Most certainly you won't wrestle with feelings of guilt afterwards.

Melatonin and Better Sleep

Melatonin is a hormone produced in the brain. This neurohormone regulates your sleep and wake cycles. Your body's internal clock controls your natural cycle of sleeping and waking hours. Melatonin is closely tied to this internal body clock. Normally, melatonin levels increase in the evening and remain high for most of the night. Conversely, melatonin levels decline in the early morning.

Sunlight affects how much melatonin the body produces. During the shorter, darker days of winter, melatonin production may be shifted a few hours from its normal time cycle. This change can lead to winter time depression symptoms commonly referred to as SAD (Seasonal Affective Disorder).

Like other hormones, melatonin levels slowly decline with age. By the age of 60, some adult bodies may produce very small amounts or none at all.

Many individuals have found supplemental melatonin to be beneficial in helping them to fall asleep faster, and remain asleep longer. The most common dosage ranges from 3.0 to 10.0 mg taken 30–60 minutes before bedtime.

Melatonin is easily found at health food stores and most grocery store vitamin aisles. It may be purchased as a solitary supplement or combined with other agents such as Magnesium, Calcium, Valerian Root, and GABA which are purported to improve the effectiveness.

Anybody deciding to try melatonin as a sleep aid should begin with a lower dose to see how it may affect them. For reasons not fully understood, people vary in their response to melatonin supplementation. Most individuals find melatonin beneficial in helping them improve sleep. Some people report no benefit whatsoever.

Melatonin is also known to have a few side effects that vary from person to person. The most prominent of these side effects is the promotion of vivid dreams. While some people find these enhanced dreams to be interesting in their complexity and detail, others report nightmares and terrifying images. For those who respond positively to it, there is little debate that melatonin can help older individuals fall asleep faster and sleep better. But you should be aware that these benefits can dramatically vary from individual to individual.

Speaking from personal experience, my wife and I both find melatonin helpful in getting a good night's sleep. Likewise, I have two friends who say they don't like to take it because it gives them nightmares and scary dream images.

Some Useful Training Products

Over the years, I have found two products very useful for regular weight training. Certainly neither of these items is a necessity, but they offer enough benefit that I personally use them all the time. If you get serious about regular training, I truly believe these products are worthy of your consideration.

Versa Gripps®

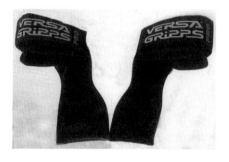 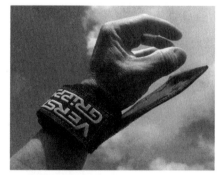

(Photo 8.8) Versa Gripps® offer protection for fingers and palms.

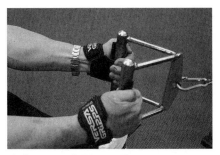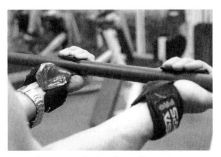

(Photo 8.9) Versa Gripps® reverse-wrapped around the bar function similarly to traditional lifting straps and remove strain on the fingers and joints when pulling heavy weights. With the black leather padding resting in the palms, protection is provided to the hands when performing pressing motions.

Many people wear standard weightlifting gloves when they go to a gym. You have no doubt seen them yourself. They are padded gloves that usually have the fingers cut off between the middle and last joint.

These types of gloves do a good job providing cushion to your palms when pressing a heavy weight, but they offer no real benefit for pulling motions. I have often wondered why they make these gloves fingerless. It seems illogical to me.

When you think about pulling against a heavy resistance, it is usually the farthest ends of your fingers that bear the brunt of the work. Yet, this is the precise spot where these standard lifting gloves offer no protection or benefit.

I play guitar. I have also been lifting weights for many years. As I passed the age of 45, I began to notice the first signs of mild pain and stiffness in the joints of my hands and fingers. This alarmed me since dexterity, flexibility, and quick mobility of the fingers is important for forming shapes on the guitar fret board.

Since my overall strength had increased over the years, it dawned on me the problem might be repeated weekly strain applied on the hands when performing heavy pulling motions.

Think about it. You may have large, wide, back muscles that can row with 150–200 lbs. But you need to hold that weight in hands that have fingers equipped with muscles not much larger than pencils.

It stands to reason that repeated working of the hands under these kinds of loads would potentially create some joint discomfort after several years. This does not even take into consideration the natural aches and pains many people begin to feel in their later years from the early stages of arthritis, or simply a half century of wear and tear on the hands.

It was around this time that I discovered Versa Gripps®. These are unique in that they act as two products in one. They offer added cushioning for the palms when performing pressing motions. More importantly for my concerns, they also work similar to the wraps used by heavy duty weight lifters and take strain off the fingers.

By reverse wrapping the gripping flap on the Versa Gripps® over the bar, the fingers are actually only used to hold the gripping flap in place. The strain of pulling or lifting is shifted away from the fingers and redirected to the full structure of the wrist and hand.

In my own case, the finger and joint discomfort I was feeling disappeared after only a few weeks. It has now been over five years since I started using these dual purpose training gloves and I rarely go to the gym without them.

If you find your fingers, joints, or knuckles aching after heavy lifting motions, these may be worth a try. In fact, their use is not limited to the gym. I know at least one person who also uses them at their job. He must carry heavy paint cans and buckets around all day. He uses these Versa Gripps® to prevent the hand pain caused by this type of repetitive lifting.

BT Burner®

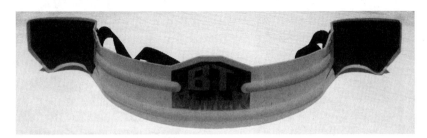

(Photo 8.10) The BT Burner® is a modern updated version of the classic Super Arm Blaster® manufactured by Joe Weider and used by famous bodybuilders of the 1970s.

If you look at any old muscle magazines from the 1970s and early 1980s you will almost certainly find photographs of bodybuilding legends like Arnold Schwarzenegger, Lou Ferrigno, Boyer Coe, Franco Columbu and others using a golden device called the "Super Arm Blaster®."

The purpose of this strap-on device was to increase focus and isolation when training biceps and triceps muscles. Although very effective at helping to build stronger arms, this is one training accessory that seemed to disappear for many years. Recently with the resurgence of old-school training methods, new improved versions of this device have become available.

The best of these new "arm blasters" is called the BT Burner®. The BT Burner® works as an arm rest and stabilizer used for performing strict bicep curls and triceps kickbacks. It provides maximum isolation on the working muscles and minimum stress on the non-working support muscles (i.e. the lower & mid back and shoulders).

This new version offers several improvements over the original 1970s model. The arm rest areas are padded near the elbows. The cutaway section for the body is deeper, allowing for the upper arms to hang in the optimum position for maximizing focus on the target muscles. The arm

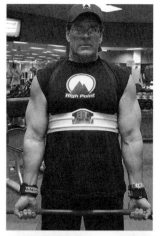

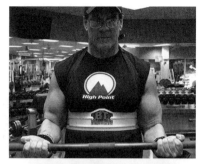

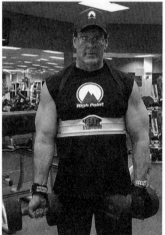

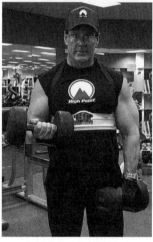

(Photo 8.11) The BT Burner® in use. This product increases the benefit and results of biceps curls and various triceps exercises.

rests are also notched, which allows for a fuller range of motion for both biceps and triceps exercises.

I always use the BT Burner® for at least one arm exercise movement on biceps and triceps days. It is very useful for helping you to maintain proper form, increase intensity on the muscle being worked, and see more results from the work you do.

A Personal View on Health Food Supplements

As a chemist, I have long held to the belief the human body is essentially a big test tube. From the day we are born, billions of chemical reactions occur in our body every day. One might say it is the slow degradation of these chemical reactions over time that produces aging, and eventual death.

With this view in mind, it could also be argued that the variables we introduce into these chemical reactions can greatly change the results. For example, a disinfecting chemical may be needed to kill germs and make water safe to drink. But what do those same chemicals that kill bacteria and virus cells do to the cells in our own bodies over years of continual exposure?

Without becoming a fanatic, I personally try to go the natural route as much as possible. For example, I try to avoid the artificial sweeteners in diet sodas, the low quality ingredients used by most fast food restaurants, and vices like tobacco, drugs, and alcohol.

When it comes to health food supplements, there are both good and bad products to be found. Without doubt there are products being sold today that have no credible research or even substantial anecdotal evidence to support their claims.

Likewise, there are many supplements such as Saw Palmetto, Glucosamine-Chondroitin-MSM, DIM, ZMA, Glutamine, Creatine, Protein powders, and others, that have an impressive track record of yielding positive benefits for millions of people. In recent years, supplements such as Saw Palmetto have come under attack by researchers who claim they have performed new studies that show no benefit from these products.

I confess I am skeptical of some of these new studies. Why am I suspicious? Some of the world's largest pharmaceutical companies have been busy the past two years buying out health supplement companies. These acquisitions have ranged from $250 million to over $1 billion in value. These are considerable purchases for companies and products that supposedly have no value or benefit.

At this same time in the Unites States, several politicians have been proposing new legislation that would change the way health food supplements are regulated and sold. As I sit writing this book, one current bill before Congress is being presented as a way to "better protect the general public."

At face value, this sounds like a well-intentioned idea. But anybody who was not born yesterday is well aware that when it comes to government, ideology does not always translate to reality. A major concern for many is the way the bill is written. The legal language used is very broad, open-ended, and subject to interpretation.

For example, this bill could allow for supplements as simple and common as multivitamins to be available by prescription only. Many Europeans are already familiar with this kind of government control. It is for this reason that so many people living in Europe use mail order to purchase their health food supplements from the United States.

Additionally, this bill would allow the FDA to make a strict list of approved vitamins, supplements, and energy drinks. Likewise, they could arbitrarily ban products that are popular and used by millions of US consumers today.

I question the real motives behind these recent actions. Certainly the intentions may be as honest and sincere as the drafters of this bill claim. Perhaps this is a genuine effort to look out for the safety of citizens. But having lived long enough to see how government and corporate partnerships tend to work in the real world, I suspect there might be something more going on.

The health food and supplement industry has shown more growth in recent years than many business sectors. The driving force behind this growth seems to be more people trying to find a way to improve their health, and ward off illness that might otherwise translate to a reliance on pharmaceutical medicines.

Some optimists believe the large pharmaceutical companies are simply looking for another income stream to diversify their product catalogs. By acquiring health food companies, they can essentially own it all—natural vitamins, supplements, and prescription drugs.

Others are concerned these acquisitions are a move to wipe out the health food industry. If pharmaceutical companies eliminate their competition via acquisition, then consumers may end up with no options except for prescription medications.

Likewise, if the Federal Government restricts and controls the sale of these products, then they can steer more people towards a restructured health industry where even a Vitamin C tablet would require a doctor's prescription. In any event, I feel this is a development worth keeping an eye on.

I can best summarize my feelings on health food products and supplements as follows: Some products are only hype with no real benefits. Other supplements have proven to be beneficial and effective.

Health foods and supplements should not be viewed as a replacement for professional medical treatment of a serious existing condition. On that same note, I feel we have become a culture obsessed with instant gratification. I believe we over-medicate ourselves by quickly looking for the "magic pill" to fix all our problems.

Modern medicine has worked wonders in helping people live a better quality of life. More importantly, modern medicine has saved lives and allowed people to live who would have otherwise perished if they had been born 100 years earlier. Even with all this in mind, there are times when reliance on medications should probably be a last resort, and not the first place we run for a solution.

The Last Words

This section marks the end of our time together.

I hope you have found the information in this book to be interesting, entertaining, and educational. More importantly, I hope you have found this to be both an inspiration and an honest roadmap for helping you to improve your level of fitness.

All my life, books have been important. I spent hundred of hours in my youth exploring the aisles of dark, dusty, used bookstores searching for hidden treasures. Much of what I learned in life came from countless hours spent reading under a shade tree in the woods or along a river bank.

For the past 50 years, I have been the lucky recipient of the knowledge books are able to give to us. Now, with the writing of this self-help guide, I hope I have made a lasting contribution to the other side of that equation. My greatest satisfaction would come from knowing this book ends up helping a multitude of people improve their fitness as they move through the second half of their lives.

All of us look back at our lives and experience moments of "Woulda, Coulda, Shoulda" regrets. If you learn from those experiences, then that is the best a mortal person can hope for.

All the days of your life that have come before this moment are like the wake of a boat. As you move forward to new adventures, those waves roll off into the distance behind you. In time, your past becomes only a story. It is today and tomorrow that define the life you are living now.

I hope you will find this book worthy of being a faithful companion as you move forward with the goal of improving your own fitness at 40, 50, 60, and beyond.

Good Luck.

Suggested Reading

For those people wishing to expand their knowledge on exercise, diet, and other self-help topics, I recommend the following books.

Recipes & Low Carb Dieting

Kress, Diane, *The Metabolism Miracle: 3 Easy Steps To Regain Control of Your Weight Permanently*. Da Capo Press, 2010.

Reno, Tosca, *The Eat-Clean Diet*. Robert Kennedy Publishing, 2006.

General Exercise & Self Help

Columbu, Franco, *Winning Bodybuilding*. Contemporary Books, 1977.

Ilardi, Dr. Stephen, *The Depression Cure: The 6 Step Program to Beat Depression without Drugs*. DaCapo Press, 2010.

Kennedy, Robert, *Bullseye: Targeting Your Life for Real Financial Wealth and Personal Fulfillment*. Robert Kennedy Publishing, 2012.

LaLanne, Jack, *Live Young Forever: 12 Steps to Optimum Health, Fitness and Longevity*. Robert Kennedy Publishing, 2009.

Reeves, Steve & Little, John & Wolff, Dr. Bob, *Building the Classic Physique: The Natural Way*. Steve Reeves International, 1995.

Wright, Dr. Vonda & Winter, Ruth, *Fitness After 40: How to Stay Strong at Any Age*. AMACOM, 2009.

Index

chest exercises for, 319–321
equipment for, 303–309
forearm exercises for, 332–334
hamstring exercises for, 338–339
leg and knee stretch, 316–317
lower back stretch, 315–316
midsection exercises for, 342–350
quadriceps exercises for, 335–338
quick reference guide for, 359
routine for, 309–311
shoulder exercises for, 321–324
shoulder rotations, 311–312
trapezius exercise for, 330–332
triceps exercises for, 324–327
warm-up for, 311
wrist rotations, 314
hormone replacement therapy (HRT), 383–384
hot flashes, 382
hydrogenation, 70–71
hyperextensions for lower back, 221–223
hypogonadism
primary, 377–378
secondary, 378–379
hypothalamus, 377

I
Ilardi, Stephen S., 390
incline barbell press, 168–169
incline dumbbell press, 169–171
injury, risk of, 2–4
insulin, 53, 56, 70, 79–81, 83, 85–86
isolation exercises, 244

J
Jamaican Jerk Chicken Tossed Salad, 123
joint health, 386
ketosis, 76
knee ups, 364–365
knees
leg and knee stretch, 162–164, 316–317
stair climbing and, 229–230

L
Lamm, Steven, 39
lat cable pulldowns, 185–187
lateral shoulder machine, 260–261
leg and knee stretch, 162–164, 316–317
leg extension warm up exercise, 198–200
leg raises, 219–221, 345–347
Leydig cells, 377
Lichten, Joanne V., 50
ligaments, 35–36
low testosterone, 39, 374–380
lower back, hyperextensions for, 221–223
lower back stretch, 161–162, 315–316
lower back tense, 365–366
L-theanine, 45, 390
lungs, 24–26
lutein, 386
lutenizing hormone (LH), 377
lying barbell triceps extensions, 268–269
lying leg curl, 205–207

Your Road to Fitness Does Not Stop Here

Visit

www.highpointproducts.com

To Continue Your Journey

- Join the Fitness Forum to chat with others. Find recipes, share your success story, discuss exercise and diet ideas that have helped others.

- Follow the Highpoint Fitness Blog to get new tips and suggestions for improving your fitness and maintaining healthy weight.

- Gear up for your new exercise lifestyle with gym bags, T-shirts, caps and BPA-free water bottles all sporting the motivational Highpoint logo.

- Email the author with your own special questions and comments.

- And more …

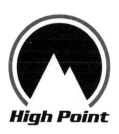

— Notes —

— Notes —

— Notes —

— Notes —

— Notes —